Diagnostic Reasoning and Treatment Decision Making in Nursing

Diagnostic Reasoning and Treatment Decision Making in Nursing

DORIS L. CARNEVALI, MN, RN
School of Nursing
University of Washington
Seattle, Washington

MARY DURAND THOMAS, PhD, RN, CS
Department of Psychosocial Nursing
University of Washington
Seattle, Washington

J. B. Lippincott Company
Philadelphia

610.73
CAR
1993

Acquisitions Editor: Donna Hilton, R.N., B.S.N.
Assistant Editor: Susan Perry
Cover Designer: Ilene Griff Design
Production Manager: Lori J. Bainbridge
Production Service: Chernow Editorial Services, Inc.
Compositor: Composing Room of Michigan, Inc.
Printer/Binder: R.R. Donnelley & Sons
Cover Printer: Lehigh Press

6 5 4 3 2

Library of Congress Cataloging-in-Publication Data

Carnevali, Doris L.
    Diagnostic reasoning and treatment decision making in nursing / Doris Carnevali, Mary Durand Thomas. — 1st ed.
        p.   cm.
    Includes bibliographical references and index.
    ISBN 0-397-54921-0
    1. Nursing—Decision making. 2. Nursing diagnosis. I. Thomas, Mary Durand. II. Title.
    [DNLM: 1. Decision Making. 2. Nursing Diagnosis. 3. Patient Care Planning. WY 100 C289d]
    RT42.C33 1993
    610.73—dc20
    DNLM/DLC
    for Library of Congress   92-49270

Any procedure or practice described in this book should be applied by the health-care practitioner under appropriate supervision in accordance with professional standards of care used with regard to the unique circumstances that apply in each practice situation. Care has been taken to confirm the accuracy of information presented and to describe generally accepted practices. However, the authors, editors, and publisher cannot accept any responsibility for errors or omissions or for consequences from application of the information in this book and make no warranty, express or implied, with respect to the contents of the book.

Every effort has been made to ensure drug selections and dosages are in accordance with current recommendations and practice. Because of ongoing research, changes in government regulations and the constant flow of information on drug therapy, reactions and interactions, the reader is cautioned to check the package insert for each drug for indications, dosages, warnings and precautions, particularly if the drug is new or infrequently used.

This book is dedicated to Dolores E. Little,
Professor Emeritus, University of Washington
School of Nursing, whose ideas, style and
generosity began the three decade clinical and
cognitive journey that resulted in this book.
And to Christine A. Tanner, Professor, School of
Nursing, Oregon Health Sciences University,
a "reformed rationalist," who was an
inspirational companion along the way.

For, however familiar and routine it may be, or seemingly unthreatening and nontragic, no nursing action or interaction that involves a patient is trivial or completely ordinary.

Renée C. Fox[1]

[1]Renée C. Fox, The Evolution of Medical Uncertainty, *Milbank Memorial Fund Quarterly/ Health and Society* 58 (1): 1–49, 1980, p. 5

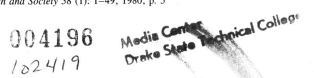

Preface

An important hallmark of professional nursing is expertise in making clinical judgments, nursing diagnoses, prognoses, and treatment decisions. It is central to effective nursing practice. These judgments and decisions emerge from the nurse's skill in attending to and processing relevant information from clinical situations. The cognitive processes and activities involved are not easily studied. As a result they have tended to remain at an implicit level in both texts and teaching. This book seeks to make explicit the thinking processes used in nursing diagnosis and treatment decisions.

Nursing process is usually regarded as consisting of four or five sequential, slightly overlapping steps. In this book the elements are shown to be highly integrated. Additionally, the step of making a clinical judgment about nursing prognosis based on prognostic data has been incorporated. This addition is introduced in Chapter 1 and discussed fully in Chapter 4. Treatment and evaluation decisions are then based, not only on diagnosis, but also on prognosis as shown in Chapter 5.

An analogy can be drawn between the cognitive processes and skills addressed in this book and such complicated skills as skiing or playing a violin. One can read and be helped to understand the mechanisms and challenges, but real learning comes in applying that knowledge and practicing those skills on varying ski slopes or on varying pieces of music of increasing complexity. In the same way, the cognitive processes and activities involved in making nursing judgments and decisions need to be understood as an initial approach. However, that is not enough. Skill needs to be developed in applying them to varying clinical situations and at varying stages of one's professional development. Exercises are suggested throughout this book to assist in application of the ideas and skills in a variety of clinical and nonclinical situations. In addition, as clinical situations are described to illustrate application of the ideas, readers are encouraged to recall patient instances or knowledge from their own experience and to add to the examples in the book in order to gain personal ownership of the content. This book requires ongoing active participation with close, consistent linkages being made between personal clinical practice and the content of the book.

Chapter 1 addresses the general nature of the tasks nurses face as they engage in nursing judgments and decisions and the ways in which the book can be used to gain insights and skills.

Chapter 2 explores the nature of memory as it affects processing of incoming stimuli and mental information. Both the limitations and richness of memory are identified as they affect the making of clinical judgments and decisions. Storage of knowledge and experience in long term memory for clinical purposes is also introduced.

Chapters 3, 4, and 5 address the cognitive processes and nursing activities involved in diagnostic reasoning, prognostic judgments, and decision making about nursing treatment. Chapter 3 examines the diagnostic reasoning process and shows how ongoing judgments during data collection are essential to final decisions. Chapter 4 looks at the nature of prognosis as it applies to the nursing domain and its relationships to other parts of the nursing process. It also examines the database needed to make prognostic judgments and the process involved. Chapter 5 considers the nature of decision making as it applies to treatment, examines both the data and knowledge needed as well as the process involved. In all three chapters involvement of the person being diagnosed or treated (whether patient or others) is encouraged, and scripts are offered to illustrate possible approaches.

Nursing judgments and decisions are not made in a vacuum. A variety of internal and external factors influence not only the judgments themselves but also their communication and implementation. Chapters 6, 7, and 8 address these factors. Chapter 6 addresses personal, environmental, and job factors that have been found to influence the activity of making clinical judgments and decisions. Chapter 7 offers one system and structure for organizing knowledge in long term memory that may improve both initial storage and access to knowledge and patient instances when they are needed in clinical practice. Chapter 8 discusses nurses' roles and role relationships associated with diagnosis and treatment planning. Roles and role relationships with patients, physicians and others are described when the nurse is carrying out delegated functions and when the nurse functions as the primary diagnostician and treatment planner in the nursing domain. Activities and behavior to enhance nurses' credibility and influence in implementation and integration of nursing judgments and treatment into the total health care plan are described.

Finally, Chapter 9 compares the differing challenges for nursing students, beginning clinicians and experienced nurses as they seek ongoing improvement of their expertise. It also provides a "road map" for the journey toward achieving excellence in these skills.

This book is intended for nursing students as well as practicing clinicians who wish to gain greater knowledge and insight into the nebulous area of thinking and information processing central to safe, effective nursing practice. Having knowledge about the processes can increase command of them.

Students.   For students the book can be used:

- In development of a personal system for structuring and storing knowledge from reading and lectures into diagnostic concepts.
- To provide guidelines for storing, retrieving, and using both patient instances and clinical knowledge in clinical courses.
- In learning how to cluster knowledge for greater efficiency in use of working memory.
- In setting patterns of practice in thinking and in use of clinical experiences to enrich knowledge.
- To increase awareness of how the environment and internal factors influence critical thinking.
- To provide guidelines for role responsibilities and behavior in interacting with others in relationship to nursing judgments and decisions.
- As an adjunct to clinical textbooks used in medical, surgical, obstetrics, pediatrics, psychiatry, community health, and subspecialty courses, etc.

Faculty.   Faculty in both classroom and clinical courses may find it helpful in:

- Developing patterns for consistently structuring knowledge in ways that facilitate systematic storage and retrieval.
- Offering ideas for objectives and learning experiences associated with cognitive processes, and role behaviors associated with the diagnostic and treatment planning processes.

Clinicians.   For nurses whose basic education did not include nursing diagnosis and treatment decision making, the book can serve as:

- An introduction and clinical guide to gaining skills.
- A guide for ongoing self-development and use of clinical practice as a learning laboratory.

For nurses whose diagnostic thinking and practices have become routine and less conscious, this book provides a reference to consult as a basis for self-evaluation. Regardless of the stage of career, one needs to value and have the capacity to periodically review and upgrade one's patterns of storage and use of nursing knowledge in judgments and decisions.

The authors invite comments and sharing of experiences in use of the ideas of the book in either clinical practice or teaching. They can be directed to Doris Carnevali at 3250 36th Ave. S.W., Seattle, WA 98126, or Mary Durand Thomas at Department of Psychosocial Nursing SC-76, University of Washington, Seattle, WA 98195.

Acknowledgments

We would like to express special gratitude to colleagues who read and commented on sections of the manuscript or who suggested resources.

Susan B. Flagler, DNS, RN
Associate Professor, Department of Parent and Child Nursing
University of Washington
Seattle, Washington

Pamela L. Jordan, PhD, RN
Associate Professor, Department of Parent and Child Nursing
University of Washington
Seattle, Washington

Jeffrey W. Thurston, MN, RN, CS
Clinical Nurse Specialist, Legal Offenders Unit
Western State Hospital
Ft. Steilacoom, Washington

Clinical Instructor, Department of Psychosocial Nursing
University of Washington
Seattle, Washington

Anne Tulk, MS, RN, CS
Clinical Nurse Specialist, Geropsychiatric Unit
Eastern State Hospital
Medical Lake, Washington

Clinical Instructor, Department of Psychosocial Nursing
University of Washington
Seattle, Washington

Vivian Wolf-Wilets, PhD, RN, FAAN
Professor, Department of Psychosocial Nursing
University of Washington
Seattle, Washington

and especially to
Christine Tanner, PhD, RN, FAAN
for her careful, expert review
of the manuscript

Doris L. Carnevali
Mary Durand Thomas

Contents

Clinical Exercises

5. Identification of patient data needed for treatment decisions beyond those used for diagnosis and prognosis
6. Analysis of influence of prognosis on treatment decisions in selected patient

Set 3   *Nursing Treatment Modalities, 136*
1. Extrapolation of nursing treatment modalities from analysis of recent nursing activities
2. Consideration of variations in a nursing diagnostic category and necessary modifications in nursing treatment
3. Comparison of different levels of severity within a nursing diagnosis and necessary modifications in nursing treatment

Set 4   *Models for Decision Making, 136*
1. Use of Decision Analysis guidelines and form in making a nursing treatment decision without and with a patient
2. Use of opportunistic thinking in making nursing treatment decisions for care of a patient
3. Use of elements of the treatment decision process in making a treatment plan for a patient
4. Critiqued practice in interacting with the patient, family, or caregiver in making treatment decisions
5. Evaluation of a treatment plan from the perspective of the elements of the treatment decision process

Set 5   *Nursing Directives, 137*
1. Precision and specificity in writing nursing directives for a selected patient using guidelines in Display 5-2
2. Evaluation of written directives as to effectiveness in guiding nursing behavior of a nursing colleague caring for this patient
3. Evaluation of nursing directives (oral and written) of other nurses as to their specificity in guiding nursing behavior
4. Purposeful contrasting of general and specific nursing directives in one's thinking

*Diagnostic
Reasoning and
Treatment Decision
Making in Nursing*

1

Nursing Diagnosis and Treatment Decision Making: Complex but Learnable Tasks

Nursing expertise is most easily recognized by what nurses do. Yet the skill in thinking that invisibly precedes the action is at least as critical as the action itself. This thinking component is not only invisible to others—even nurses themselves may be less than fully aware that it is occurring. Once nurses become expert in nursing diagnosis and treatment of particular phenomena or situations, this important act of thinking can become second nature—without really being aware of it. Beginning nurses too often do not realize that they are "treating" patients using attitudes and actions based on subtle nursing judgments. Recognized or not, these clinical judgments and decisions are a part of professional nursing practice.

What Are Nursing Diagnoses?

In the proceedings of their ninth conference, the North American Nursing Diagnosis Association (NANDA) defined a nursing diagnosis as:

> A clinical judgment about an individual, family, or community response to actual or potential health problems/life processes which provides the basis for definitive therapy toward achievement of outcomes for which the nurse is accountable.
>
> (Carpenito, 1991, p. 65, citing NANDA Board of Directors and the Taxonomy Committee)

In this book, the focus for nursing diagnosis is expanded somewhat to include the context of daily living within which the responses occur and external resources that affect the individual, family, or community. Given this approach, diagnoses, such as impaired gas exchange, decreased cardiac output, or knowledge deficit, would be integrated with the diagnosed requirements of daily living that have to be met and the identified external resources that help or hinder in the situation. For example:

> One person with impaired gas exchange or decreased cardiac output may be in a hospital with adequate staffing and technology to assist with physical demands and may have a supportive family. Another person with a comparable deficit may live at home (or be homeless), with or without the benefit of a caregiver. The contextual demands of daily living on the individual and the status of external resources can vary widely, creating the need for differing nursing diagnoses and certainly different nursing treatments.

In essence, the perspective is diagnosing of the status of the balance between requirements placed on the person or group being diagnosed and the functional capacities and external resources for meeting those requirements within the context of the presenting health situation. Thus, not only is the word *response* used in conjunction with nursing diagnosis, but also *situation*—the context surrounding the person and the responses.

Nursing diagnoses result from a series of clinical judgments. Clinical judgments are complex decisions about the status of the individual or family and the contextual situation affecting the person's or family's responses based on findings and their interpretation. Characteristics of clinical judgment contribute to its complexity. These include uncertainty, variability in clinical situations, availability of data, ambiguity of data, and their value-laden nature. Clinical judgments incorporate several types of judgments including:

- *Perceptual judgments* on what data to collect, whether a sign or symptom is present or not, what strengths and positive elements exist in the person and contextual situation.
- *Inferential judgments* on the meaning and significance of the findings as well as relationships existing among the collected data.
- *Diagnostic judgments* as to whether any clusters of cues exist that fit patterns associated with particular diagnoses   (Gordon, 1987).

Several theoretical frameworks have been developed to explain the nature of cognitive and observation processes involved in making clinical judgments. Tanner (1983) described various theoretical frameworks for approaching clinical judgment (see also references on theories of clinical judgment at the end of this chapter). This book will use information processing theory.

Nurses' clinical judgments result in cognitive products, either nonverbalized impressions or formal diagnoses. When a nursing diagnosis is formalized, it has a consistent structure containing two or three components:

- an identified potential or existing health state, health problem, condition, or life process;
- related factors; and occasionally,
- responses to the problem.

Clinical impressions or diagnoses are crucial in that they become the basis for viewing the patient and determining nursing treatment.

Risks Associated with Nursing Diagnosis

Nursing diagnoses are the diagnostician's interpretation, abstraction, and representation of the reality of the patient's or family's experiences, responses, and situation. Sometimes these nursing judgments take on a life of their own and become more real for nurses than the actual experiences taking place for the individual, family, or group. Then one tends to view patients from the perspective of the diagnosis, e.g., ineffective in individual or family coping, impaired in their social interactions, dysfunctional in their grieving. When the diagnoses are *currently* correct, they are helpful in guiding observation and planning definitive nursing treatment. There is always a possibility that the diagnosis was not an accurate representation, e.g., it represented a nurse's value system but did not take into account the patient's or family's norms, values, or beliefs about coping, interacting, or grieving (Chrisman, 1991). Or the diagnosis may have been correct initially, but the situation and responses have changed and the diagnosis has not been updated. Then the mind-set and the basis for treatment are no longer valid. In addition, as an abstraction, some meaning inevitably is lost.

Thus it is important to acknowledge the difference between the reality and its representation in nursing diagnosis. There is no question that nursing diagnosis contributes to effective nursing practice. However, nurses need to maintain an awareness that the diagnosis is only a label or categorization for what a person is experiencing.

Nursing Diagnoses and Treatment Decisions Are Important

Nursing judgments about patients and the subsequent treatments may not seem as dramatic as some medical diagnoses and treatments. Yet the well-being of patients and families can be supported in significant ways by accurate nursing diagnoses and effective treatment or disrupted by incorrect nursing diagnosis and treatment. Any practicing nurse can recall situations in which nursing diagnosis and treatment made a major positive or negative difference in a patient's well-being.

Not only is it important that nurses diagnose prior to treatment, but the accuracy and quality of those diagnoses need to be good or the treatment may be ineffective, and even harmful. A nurse's failure to attend to relevant, available data during the diagnostic process can result in a failure to identify a potential or existing problem. Treatment will be neither planned nor implemented because the problem area was not recognized. A nurse can incorrectly interpret data, develop an incorrect diagnosis, and therefore prescribe incorrectly for the wrong phenomenon. A nurse can make a vague or general diagnosis when data are available to make a specific one, with the result that treatment will not be individualized and thus be potentially less effective. A nurse can stereotype—presume data to be present when they are not. Treatment will then be directed to a phenomenon that may or may not exist.

Treatment decisions made with or without awareness depend on some prior judgment about patient status and situation. Those judgments need to be rigorous and accurate if treatment is to be maximally therapeutic.

Nursing Diagnoses Are Complex and Transitory

Some nurses have suggested that nursing diagnosis and treatment planning should be made simple. However, human beings, their responses to health-related conditions, and their situations are not simple.

Complexity in Nursing Diagnosis and Treatment Planning

While many human responses to health conditions and situations have enough commonalities to lend themselves to diagnosis, they also can show a high degree of variability. No two patients, even those suffering from the same pathology, respond to the illness and health care experience in the same way. No two healthy individuals, for whom health promotion would be the goal, approach health promotion and maintenance in the same way. Furthermore, at times the manifestations of any given response may be muted or distorted, so data for making clinical judgments may be hard to notice. This does not begin to cover additional factors nurses need to consider such as: the support systems available to the individual and family, and demands being made on them as a result of the context within which the health or illness experience is being managed. Contextual factors include past and current patterns of daily living in the community or institutional setting, values and beliefs, role responsibilities, family or caregivers, status of external resources (Carnevali and Reiner, 1990; Carnevali and Patrick, 1993). Because nursing's clientele is so complex, there is no way to make diagnosis and treatment of health-related responses and situations simple without being unrealistic. *Simple diagnoses for complex situations do not lead to effective treatment.*

Transiency in Nursing Diagnosis and Treatment Planning

An additional factor adding to complexity in nursing diagnosis and treatment planning is the reality that human responses and situations are dynamic—they do not stay the same. Thus a diagnosis and treatment plan that may be accurate and therapeutic at one point in time may be inaccurate and inappropriate in a matter of hours or days, certainly in weeks.

Both rapidly and slowly occurring changes bring their own complexity to nursing diagnosis. Managing to stay abreast of diagnostic and treatment planning tasks with rapidly changing patient status and circumstances is a challenge. Often this occurs in hectic and demanding emergency, critical, and acute care situations. Conversely, diagnosis in relatively stable states brings its own difficulties. It is not easy to maintain "fresh eyes" and to attend to subtle changes in individuals or groups who change slowly. Neither is it easy to translate these minichanges into accurate and precise diagnoses that will result in appropriately modified treatment plans. Further, the settings in which nurses regularly care for a stable clientele usually require heavy caseloads, so there is less contact time within which to notice small but significant changes.

Both the complexity of health-related areas that nurses are required to diagnose and the reality that nursing diagnoses are much less stable than medical diagnoses make diagnosing and treatment planning challenging tasks in nursing. Nevertheless, professional nursing requires that nursing clinicians be as skilled and rigorous in these cognitive skills as other health-care professionals whom the public pays to assist in its health care management. Diagnostic and treatment planning expertise in complex, changing patient situations is essential to professional nursing practice.

Gaining Expertise in Diagnostic Reasoning and Treatment Planning Is Doable

Gaining expertise in diagnostic and treatment decisions is neither a quick nor an easy task. On the other hand, gaining expertise in recognizing and diagnosing patient situations in the field of nursing is doable. These are skills that can be learned. They can be learned, in part, from reading and from others. Ultimately, however, working expertise will emerge from personally seeking to learn in one's clinical encounters with patients and colleagues. Like skiing or playing a violin, expertise is achieved by doing it, over and over, and by being consistently evaluative of one's performance. Conversely, ineffective performance can be reinforced by repeated incorrect or sloppy practice.

Diagnostic Reasoning and Treatment Planning Expertise Grows Slowly

These are slow-growing skills, not accomplished in a week or a month, or even a school year. In Chapter 2, on memory, the reader will see that growing skill in making diagnostic and treatment decisions is dependent on theoretical knowledge, clinical knowledge, and storage of specific patient instances. Gaining expertise also depends on repeated application of one's observational and cognitive skills during encounters with a growing number of patients and their situations in the course of one's clinical experience.

Gaining Diagnostic–Treatment Planning Expertise Can Be Enjoyable

While gaining expertise in the use of knowledge and skills can be demanding, it need not be dull. Using patient encounters as a basis for professional growth can be an ongoing adventure. Each patient-family[1] situation produces new challenges. For the nurse who is seeking to learn, each clinical encounter offers the opportunity to recognize familiar commonalities, to see new variations, and to better prepare for another clinical encounter. There is little occasion to become bored. Like any

---

[1]In this book family is described as a small social system of individuals that persists over years and decades linked by affections and loyalties and living in one or more households (Terkelsen, 1980); or, the person or group of people identified by the patient as "family."

advanced skill, there is no endpoint where one can cognitively ease off and say, "Now I've arrived; I can just sit back and take it easy."

Opportunities for Gaining Expertise Are Almost Unlimited

The nurse's work setting, whether used by a student or a nurse, provides almost unlimited opportunities to practice and gain expertise in diagnosis and treatment planning. The observation and thinking associated with diagnosis and treatment of nursing problems are clinically grounded, oriented to the reality of the patient's situation. The taking in and cognitive processing of information is pervasive, taking place in most patient, family, or group encounters.

Wide-ranging Focus

Nursing diagnosis and treatment planning are wide-ranging. Targets for nursing diagnoses and treatment vary widely. While there is almost always a central individual, often a person in a patient role, the nurse frequently has responsibility for others who are critical to this person's capacity to manage the health situation. Thus, they too may be a focus for diagnosis and treatment. Typically, they include the caregivers, family members of any age, or others who closely share the person's health experience and who affect patient outcomes.

Variability in Status of Those Being Diagnosed and Treated

Because nursing deals with human responses to actual or potential health issues, nurses' diagnostic and treatment thinking covers a broad range. The health-related areas being addressed involve individuals and families having quite differing situations. They may be healthy or ill, and may range in age from the newborn to the elderly. The person's health situation may involve any of the medical clinical specialties. The nurse may enter the person's health world at any point in time from a health promotion stage, at the beginning of an illness or at any stage in a disease process, including dying. Where trauma or disease is involved, the projected course of events may be acute or chronic, rapidly changing or stable.

Variations in Settings for Nursing Diagnosis and Treatment Planning

The setting within which nursing diagnosis and treatment are done affects the process. These settings can be quite different from each other and can influence one's diagnostic and treatment practices. Nursing diagnosis and treatment may occur in the home, ambulatory care clinics, schools, work places, senior citizen centers, rehabilitation centers, and at various levels of critical or acute care, long-term care, and hospice care.

Summary

It can be seen that opportunities to gain skill in diagnosing and treatment planning are ever-present. For the creative nurse, even if limited to one work setting, it is possible to encounter a variety of individuals and groups who can benefit from nursing's expertise as they seek to manage their health-related daily living. One can continue to gain skill in situations reflecting a variety of considerations. Nursing offers both richness and variety in learning experiences for the student or nurse who truly seeks increasing expertise.

This book takes into account the wide-ranging clinical nature of nursing diagnosis and treatment planning. In order to realistically demonstrate the processes in nursing practice and to ground them in clinical situations, readers will find many of the ideas illustrated by clinical examples. Additionally, the exercises at the end of process-oriented chapters show readers how to use clinical encounters to practice the skills and test or critique the ideas.

Personal Watchbirds: Creation, Feeding, Training, and Use

Much of the work of gaining expertise in diagnosis and treatment is associated with personal clinical practice. Therefore, it becomes important to develop some usable, enjoyable strategies for *critical self-awareness* of one's cognitive behavior, judgments, and decisions. Some nurses find this ongoing awareness and analysis of cognitive strategies a comfortable activity. Others have been helped by creation of an externalized "observer." One strategy for making this self-analysis more concrete is suggested in the book. It is the creation and use of a personal watchbird.

The idea is to create an image of a bird to one's own liking—one that seems compatible as a professional companion. The imagery should be quite concrete and complete. It should include the kind of bird—its size, features, coloring, and personality—perhaps even a name. Figure 1-1 illustrates the watchbird that has evolved for the authors.

Ours is a small owl, named Socrates for its capacity to ask questions that lead to logical conclusions. It has an owl's large eyes and a capacity to turn its head easily in order to take note of the entire situation. Its coloring is unobtrusive. Socrates is alert and ready to notice how the owner is observing, thinking, and acting but is also a rather gentle bird. Socrates has been known to take a nip at the owner when a particularly serious gaffe is about to be or has been made but, on the whole, gives feedback in a nonthreatening way. Socrates is willing to regularly ingest knowledge and experience and, when instructed, will use that knowledge to observe or to help critically analyze a situation. Over time Socrates has become a valued companion in the ongoing task of self-analysis and self-improvement in diagnosis and treatment decisions.

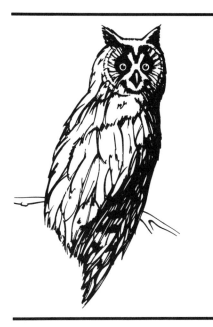

FIGURE 1-1   "Socrates," an Example of a Personal Watchbird

The creation of a personal watchbird is discussed in this first chapter because readers may find it useful to create, feed, and train their watchbirds in the course of reading the book. One can read about a particular activity or idea and feed it to the watchbird (store it for self-awareness and self-analysis), and then plan how to use it to observe thinking or behavior in the clinical setting. In the exercises the reader or the watchbird may be trained or instructed as to what to observe and the kind of feedback that will be useful during and after the activity.

A New Look at Nursing Process

In this book the traditional nursing process model (assessment, diagnosis, planning, intervention, and evaluation) has been modified. The revised version used is shown in Figure 1-2.[2]

It can be seen that data collection (assessment) and diagnosis are combined in an integrated first step. The reasoning behind this modification is covered in Chapter 3. A new step has been added addressing the tasks of collecting prognostic data and making prognostic judgments, as discussed in Chapter 4. Both diagnostic and prognostic judgments serve as a foundation for planning treatment. Data from the

[2]For the reader's convenience, the figure appears again in Chapter 4.

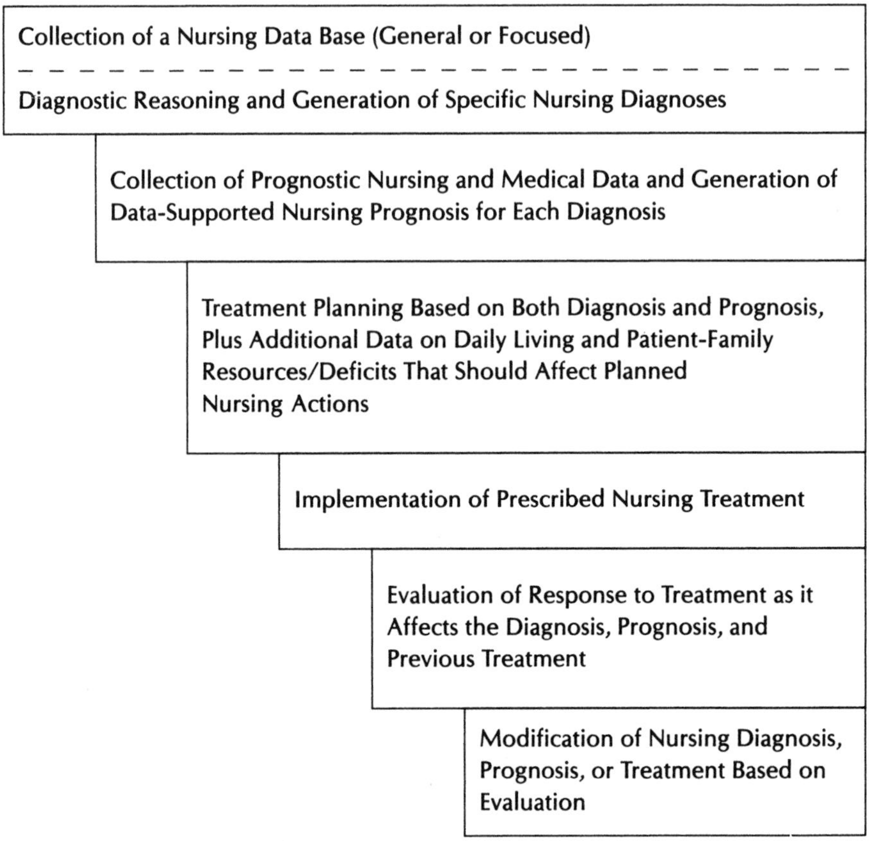

Collection of a Nursing Data Base (General or Focused)
- -
Diagnostic Reasoning and Generation of Specific Nursing Diagnoses

Collection of Prognostic Nursing and Medical Data and Generation of Data-Supported Nursing Prognosis for Each Diagnosis

Treatment Planning Based on Both Diagnosis and Prognosis, Plus Additional Data on Daily Living and Patient-Family Resources/Deficits That Should Affect Planned Nursing Actions

Implementation of Prescribed Nursing Treatment

Evaluation of Response to Treatment as it Affects the Diagnosis, Prognosis, and Previous Treatment

Modification of Nursing Diagnosis, Prognosis, or Treatment Based on Evaluation

FIGURE 1-2   Nursing Process as It Incorporates Nursing Prognosis

patient and contextual situation are added to formulate the individualized treatment plan. A final step has been added that explicitly identifies the task of using evaluative data to modify earlier judgments and decisions associated with treatment, prognosis, or diagnosis.

Using This Book for Professional Growth

This book seeks to address the cognitive processes involved in making clinical judgments leading to diagnosis, prognosis, and treatment decisions. The insights could prove helpful in developing strategies and patterns of observation and processing of information for the beginner, as well as for the nurse who has become somewhat automatic in these processes.

There is no question that these processes are complex. Therefore, the book may best be used in small sections. Read the outline preceding each chapter to gain a sense of the chapter's flow, then read the chapter to gain an overview. Finally, select one section. Read it. Think about it. There are many clinical examples. In addition, it is suggested that the reader personally seek out or recall examples in order to parallel the activity being illustrated. Do not be satisfied with just one. Think of or search for several that reflect a variety of situations and patient states, or several in which the patient status was similar but the responses, daily living, and external resources varied. Learning in this book will be most effective if the content is used primarily as a springboard for your own initiative and efforts.

References

CARNEVALI D, PATRICK M: *Nursing Management for the Elderly,* 3rd ed. Philadelphia: J.B. Lippincott, 1993.

CARNEVALI D, REINER A: *The Cancer Experience: Nursing Diagnosis and Management.* Philadelphia: J.B. Lippincott, 1990.

CARPENITO L: The NANDA definition of nursing diagnosis, pp. 65–71. In Carroll-Johnson RM (ed): *Classification of Nursing Diagnoses: Proceedings of the Ninth Conference.* Philadelphia: J.B. Lippincott, 1991.

CHRISMAN N: Culture-sensitive nursing care. pp. 34–47. In Patrick M, Woods S, Craven R, Rokosky J, Bruno P (eds): *Medical–Surgical Nursing: Pathophysiological Concepts,* 2nd ed. Philadelphia: J.B. Lippincott, 1991.

GORDON M: *Nursing Diagnosis: Process and Application,* 2nd ed. New York: McGraw-Hill, 1987.

Tanner C: Research on clinical judgment. In Holzemer WM (ed): *Review of Research in Nursing Education.* Thorofare, NJ: Slack, 1983.

TERKELSEN K: Toward a theory of the family life cycle. In Carter E, McGoldrick M (eds): *The Family Life Cycle: A Framework for Family Therapy.* New York: Gardner Press, 1980.

Additional Readings on Theories of Clinical Judgment

Decision Theory

ALBERT DA: Decision theory in medicine: A review and critique. *Health and Society* 56:362–401, 1978.

HAMMOND KR, HURSCH CJ, TODD FJ: Analyzing the components of clinical inference. *Psychological Review* 71:438–456, 1964.

HAMMOND KR, KELLY KJ, SCHNEIDER RJ, VANCINI M: Clinical inferences in nursing. *Nursing Research,* 13: Spring, Summer, and Fall issues, 1966.

KELLY KJ: An approach to the study of clinical inference in nursing: Part III. Utilization of the "Lens Model" method to study the inferential process of the nurse. *Nursing Research* 13:319–322, 1966.

Information Processing Theory

ELSTEIN AS, SHULMAN LS, SPRAFKA SA: *Medical Problem-Solving: An Analysis of Clinical Reasoning.* Cambridge, MA: Harvard University Press, 1978.

NEWELL A, SHAW JD, SIMON HA: Elements of a theory of human problem-solving. *Psychological Review* 65:151–166, 1958.

NEWELL A, SIMON HA: *Human Problem Solving.* Englewood Cliffs, NJ: Prentice-Hall, 1972.

SIMON HA: Information processing theory of human problem solving. In Estes WK (ed): *Handbook of Cognitive Process Vol 5: Human Information Processing.* Hillsdale, NJ: Erlbaum Assoc., 1978.

Phenomenologic Approach

BENNER P: *From Novice to Expert: Power and Excellence in Nursing Practice.* Palo Alto, CA: Addison-Wesley, 1984.

DREYFUS SE, DREYFUS HL: *A Five-Stage Model of the Mental Activities Involved in Directed Skill Acquisition.* Berkeley, CA: University of California, 1980.

HEIDEGGER M: *Being and Time.* (J MacQuarrie and E Robinson, trans.). New York: Harper & Row, 1962 (original work published in 1927).

PYLES SH, STERN PN: Discovery of nursing gestalt in critical care nursing: The importance of the gray gorilla syndrome. *Image: The Journal of Nursing Scholarship* 15(2):51–57, 1983.

2

Memory in Clinical Judgments and Decisions

Making diagnostic judgments and treatment decisions involves taking in information from patients and their environments, processing that information, classifying it, and making decisions for action. These clinical cognitive activities require use of three types of memory currently described in the literature—sensory memory, short term/working memory, and long term memory. Understanding the nature of these three forms of memory and the factors affecting them may enable clinicians to more effectively use memory resources available to them.

Sensory Memory

Sensory memory is the portion of memory that receives stimuli from the external and internal world via the senses (see Figure 2-1). It has great capacity to receive stimuli but is able to retain only a small portion in the actual memory system.

The function of sensory memory is thought to be that of providing guaranteed persistence at the onset of a stimulus, thus insuring the perception system a minimum time to process incoming stimuli (Coltheart, 1983). Stimuli storage time in sensory memory is very short. Visual stimuli are automatically held up to a half second. Speech sounds are retained no longer than 2–3 seconds (Ashcraft, 1989, p. 51). While only auditory and visual sensory memory have been studied, it is assumed that the other senses pass through a comparable sensory memory. There

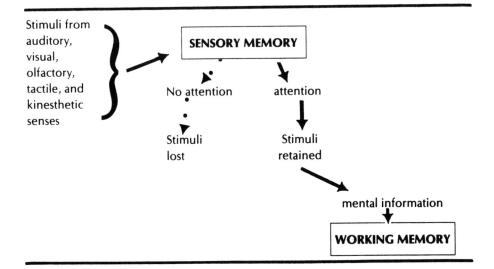

FIGURE 2-1   Sensory Memory

is some indication that it is possible to hold both visual and auditory stimuli in sensory memory a little longer to assure that processing is possible (Baddeley, 1990, p. 37).

During these milliseconds cognitive processes related to **attention** and initial **encoding** must act on the stimuli in order to send them on to working memory for further action. Encoding in sensory memory involves the initial basic *transforming of incoming sensations into mental representations* or *interpretations* of those sensations. For example:

The sounds coming into the ears from the stethoscope can be encoded as:
lub-dup lub-dup   or   lub-dup *ta*   or   *ta* lub-dup,

The sensation of intermittent pressure on finger tips placed over the radial artery can be encoded as radial pulse.

Visual stimuli of certain peaks on an ECG tracing could be encoded as an ST wave.

Olfactory stimuli from a patient's breath might be encoded as fetid, sweet and fruity, or smelling of tobacco or alcohol.

The combined absence of sound and the sight of an unwavering needle moving to lower numbers on a sphygmomanometer dial, followed by a sound of *"dub dub"* and corresponding pulsation of the needle on a dial number could be encoded as systolic blood pressure.

If attending and processing do not occur, the information is lost, to be replaced by other incoming stimuli.

The sensory memory of a nurse engaged in diagnosis and treatment planning receives innumerable stimuli. Some of these will be irrelevant or unimportant in terms of nursing diagnosis; others will be highly significant. Only those stimuli given attention will be available for further processing, the remainder will be lost.

The experienced nurse attends to stimuli considered to be relevant. Relevance, in turn, can be linked to one's specialization. A clinical specialist in respiratory care is more likely to attend to stimuli associated with the respiratory system, while a psychiatric nurse specialist may be more attuned to cues of a psychosocial nature. Each could lose significant cues if attention is paid only to stimuli within a personal field of specialization.

Learning which incoming stimuli warrant attention is a part of professional development. Discipline-specific learning initially comes through classroom experiences and reading as well as earlier life experiences. It is developed and sharpened, however, through repeated clinical experiences—becoming aware of times when significant cues were kept and used and times when cues should have been retained but were not noticed. It is one of the elements of growing diagnostic expertise.

See *Exercise Set 1* for activities dealing with sensory memory.

Working Memory

Short term memory has been the traditional name for that portion of memory holding current information and information that has received recent attention. The term is being replaced by *working memory* (WM) to more accurately describe the activities taking place in this part of the memory system (Baddeley, 1981). See Figure 2-2. In contrast to sensory memory that receives environmental stimuli, WM receives information from the internal, mental world. Working memory is the next destination for information passed along from sensory memory, but it receives input

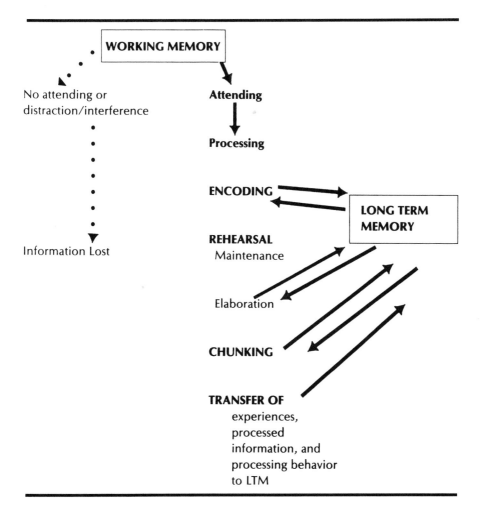

FIGURE 2-2 Working Memory

from long term memory as well. WM depends on sound and pronunciation codes but also stores visual information, verbal information, and information on physical movement. It has a limited capacity of 5–9 chunks[1] of data (Miller, 1956). Information can be held in WM for a relatively short time (15–20 seconds) unless mental repetition or other processing takes place. Information in WM is easily lost as a result of interference from other incoming information or distraction in the environment.

Description of Working Memory

Because working memory is the memory system component where active processing of information occurs, it has been likened to:

- A "scratch pad" where the results of intermediate processing are "scribbled" for later use (Ashcraft, 1989, pp. 54–55).
- A "blackboard" where the mind performs computations and posts partial results (Waldorp, 1987, p. 1565).
- The mind's information processor that takes information "on the fly," interprets it immediately and lets unneeded information fall away to make room for more input (Just and Carpenter, 1980).
- An executive control system in charge of devoting conscious processing resources to other components of the memory system (Salame and Baddeley, 1982).

All of these suggest a system for both temporarily holding and actively processing information.

Activities in Working Memory

Several cognitive activities take place in working memory. These include **encoding,**[2] **rehearsal, recoding/chunking,** and **transfer of information to and from long term memory** (Craik and Lockhart, 1972). Since these activities affect diagnostic thinking, it may help to look more closely at each of them.

Encoding/Interpretation

The initially encoded bits of mental information coming in from sensory memory are further processed by assigning more precise meaning or interpretation to them.

---

[1]A "chunk" is a piece of mental information consisting of one or more units of related information that has become familiar from earlier repeated encounters. It is recognized as a single unit (Larkin, McDermott, Simon & Simon, 1980).

[2]Encoding is the term cognitive scientists use to describe the transforming of incoming stimuli into mental information that then is available for additional refinement and further mental processing. Nurses are more likely to identify the level of encoding done in working memory as interpretation or assignment of meaning.

They are encoded into a form that promotes the activities taking place in WM. The examples below identify some types of encoding that can occur in WM for clinicians in the nursing field.

Heart Sounds

Encoded sounds transmitted via stethoscope to the ears and sensory memory as:

WM (assigns more precise meaning or interpretation):

lub-dup lub-dup	normal heart sound
lub-dup-*ta*	ventricular gallop
ta-lub-dup	atrial gallop

(Underhill, 1991, p. 625)

Pulse

Information from sensory memory as pulsations of the radial artery.

WM encodes as "radial pulse" but can be more richly and precisely encoded in terms of:

Rate
Number of pulsations per minute.

Rhythm
Pattern of pulsations, e.g., regular/irregular (rhythmic arrhythmia/arrhythmic arrhythmia).

Volume

   0   Not palpable
 +1   Thready, weak, difficult to find, can be obliterated by exerting pressure
 +2   Can be located only with light pressure of fingers, but once located, can be felt
 +3   Easily found, pressure on finger remains constant—does not fade in and out; Intermittent pulsations continue despite increasing pressure from fingers
 +4   Strong, bounding, easily felt, cannot be obliterated with pressure from fingers

(Wild, Craven, and Cunningham, 1991, p. 804)

The way in which encoding occurs is important. Using language to encode is one effective strategy. Linking the new information into systematic relations with previous knowledge is another.

Encoding precisely the many distinctive features (as illustrated in the radial pulse example above) has been found to help in subsequent discrimination (Moscovitch and Craik, 1976; Baddeley, 1990). Seeking richness, detail, and precision in encoding or interpretation leads to better performance.

Encoding can be a conscious process with unfamiliar stimuli but can become automatic with multiple repetitions and continued experience. Accuracy and precision in encoding stimuli associated with one's professional practice is one dimension of clinical expertise and a necessary element of diagnostic reasoning and treatment decision making. Encoding expertise in WM involves recognition of information from sensory memory and adequate professional language or imagery to further encode them.

Rehearsal

Rehearsal is a mental recycling activity serving to retain stimuli in WM. There are two types of rehearsal activity: *maintenance* and *elaboration* (Craik and Watkins, 1973).

Maintenance rehearsal is the activity of simply repeating information in order to retain it a bit longer in WM. For example:

A nurse is at the patient's bedside and is gathering data on vital signs but does not have paper and pen to make a notation. In order to retain the numbers until they can be documented on the patient's record at the desk, the nurse "rehearses" them several times.

Elaborative rehearsal is a process of reorganizing new information using the information's meaning to help store and remember it (Ashcraft, 1989; Baddeley, 1990, p. 172). It elaborates on the item representation by drawing relationships between what is already known (LTM) and information currently being processed. It is an activity used to transfer material from working memory to long term memory. For example:

A patient who is in the terminal stage of disease has recently given cues signaling awareness that death is probably imminent. In encountering this patient several times today, the nurse receives conflicting cues. At some times the patient speaks of expecting to die soon and at other times of feeling improved and expecting to get well. Given the nurse's present concept of grieving, the expectation was that once a loss had been initially accepted, the person would no longer vacillate back to denial or uncertainty.

Cues sent by this patient conflict with the concept in the nurse's long term memory. The nurse incorporates the newly encountered grieving responses into the concept of grief work in semantic long term memory and stores the experiences of this variant patient situation in episodic long term memory.[3]

The next time the nurse encounters a person in transition from the denial phase of grief work, her knowledge will also include the possibility of vacillation.

---

[3]A description of long term memory, including episodic, semantic, and production memory follows, beginning on p. 23.

This second, more demanding type of rehearsal is hypothesized to result in greater long term learning. Elaborative rehearsal, like encoding, involves semantics and linkage to knowledge and experiences already stored in long term memory.

Recoding/Chunking

Earlier it was noted that working memory has a limited capacity of 5–9 chunks. One way to increase that capacity is to recode information by grouping related items together and then remembering the newly formed group as one item. A chunk may contain one item of information or many related items. The goal is to make the chunks meaningful and as easily retrievable as possible—usually by assigning a recognition tag or label such as "respirations." For example:

A beginning nursing student may observe respirations and have only one item in the chunk—rate: 24/min.

An experienced nurse might have a "respiratory chunk" containing the following items after observing a patient's breathing: 24/min, prolonged expiratory phase, elevated shoulders, pursed lip breathing, using sternocleidomastoid and scalene muscles to aid breathing, sitting with elbows on knees, hyperresonance to percussion, diminished breath sounds on auscultation.

As seen in the preceding example, chunks may contain items related to one body system. A chunk may also be clustered around response to a particular situation. For example:

Subjective data: reports having been awakened from her sleep by a man in her bedroom . . . fought him off and sustained a few bruises . . . afraid to sleep because of recurrent nightmares . . . 3+ anxiety when left alone in the house . . . unable to concentrate . . . flits from one task to another . . . occasionally finds herself outside in the yard and then remembers having heard a noise in the house . . . checks to see that doors and windows are locked many times/day . . . poor concentration . . . thinks she recognizes the intruder as someone who lives nearby . . . feels panic and anger when she sees him . . . drives to the market now instead of walking for fear of meeting him. Tag: posttrauma response.

Forming these "enriched units" initially requires some difficult mental effort (Ashcraft, 1989, p. 142). However, repeated experience with comparable situations can cause chunking to become more automatic. For example, nurses on a respiratory disease unit would routinely have large chunks of information on breathing patterns while nurses on a posttrauma stress unit or rape clinic would chunk a full array of immediate and delayed responses to the experience of personal trauma.

Transfer of Information to Long Term Memory

An important function of WM is transmission of information to long term memory. Three types of information are transferred:

- The experience itself to episodic memory.
- Knowledge (new or previously experienced) about the experience to semantic memory to either modify or reinforce previously stored concepts or lists or to create new ones.
- The experience of processing, retrieving, and transferring activities to episodic memory or to an area identified sometimes as "production memory"—memory of "how to's" (Anderson, 1985).

These three types of information storage increase efficiency in subsequent encounters with situations similar to earlier experiences. For example, the nurse who encountered a patient vacillating in acknowledgment of her impending death could have stored the experience and knowledge in long term memory. In subsequent experiences with dying patients she might:

Remember the instance of the patient who vacillated between hope and acceptance of death within a period of hours and thus consider this possibility the next time she cares for someone who is dying.

Remember the experience of satisfaction or dissatisfaction with her own response and consider possible modifications in her nursing actions.

Recall the signs and symptoms that manifested the vacillation response when retrieving the concept of grieving from semantic memory.

This nurse might also have done some additional reading on grief work and uncertainty to gain more knowledge about the dynamics, manifestations, and nursing treatment of terminally ill patients. The actual experiences of encoding, chunking, linking with long term memory, and assigning meaning are stored in episodic and production memory where skill and speed can be built into subsequent information processing in similar future situations.

Skilled Memory

One other term has been applied to the working memory structure—that is **skilled memory.** It is suggested that many repetitions of linkages between working memory and long term memory can lead to a rapid, automatic interaction between the two parts of the system. Recent research using positron emission tomography (PET) also suggests that visual stimuli (and presumably other stimuli) leave a trace in the brain, so that when the same stimuli are presented again, less neural activity is required to process it (Squire et al., 1992). When this level of neural efficiency occurs, there is a blurring of the two parts of the memory system and one is said to have developed **skilled memory** (Ericsson, Chase, and Faloon, 1980).

Skilled memory emerges when experts in a particular field learn how to build efficient, often complicated, organizational systems for storing information in long term memory. Repeated practice in using these networks permits the expert to shuffle information in and out of long term memory so quickly that, in areas of expertise, long term memory becomes an extension of working memory (Waldorp, 1987).

In nursing we undoubtedly see skilled memory in use among experienced nurses who often need much less patient data in order to recognize the diagnosis because the patient data have been quickly augmented by information from long term memory involving experience with, and knowledge of, similar instances.

See *Exercise Set 2* for activities dealing with working memory.

Long Term Memory

Long term memory (LTM) is that part of the memory system capable of holding information for longer than seconds or minutes; in fact it seems to be able to store unlimited amounts of material indefinitely. There is apparently little forgetting in LTM, only difficulty in access and retrieval. Long term memory receives information from and transmits information to working memory as shown in Figure 2-3.

Long term memory has been divided into two subcategories: episodic and semantic (Tulving, 1972). Episodic memory stores personal experiences; semantic memory is the permanent repository for knowledge, concepts and language. Episodic and semantic memory are highly interactive, and there is ongoing controversy as to whether they indeed are separate (Ashcraft, 1989, p. 358; Baddeley, 1990, p. 378; Bruner, Goodnow and Austin, 1956). However, there does seem to be general acceptance that human beings do store two different types of information—personal experiences and knowledge—and that these are different forms of information. Separating them seems to be a useful conceptualization for this book at this point in time.

Certainly in nursing it is important to differentiate between a personal experience and general knowledge. Diagnosis and treatment planning based solely on personal experience could be dangerous. The number of experiences could be few, atypical, and perhaps subject to distortion in recall. On the other hand, theoretical knowledge, stored in semantic memory without the addition of memories of personal clinical experience, also can produce ineffective diagnosis and treatment planning (Schmidt, Norman, and Boshuizen, 1990). Each nurse's diagnosis and treatment planning is based on a combination of experiential memory and acquired knowledge, both prior to and after entering the professional role. Obviously then, each nurse has different episodic memories to retrieve. For example:

Nurses may have had differing experiences with anxiety and attitudes toward it.

Professionally, a pediatric nurse will recall responses to anxiety among children of different ages facing treatments that threaten them. Psychiatric nurses will recall the behavior and situations of psychotic individuals suffering from anxiety states. Personal and clinical experiences with anxiety will differ from one nurse to another, thus their episodic memories will be different.

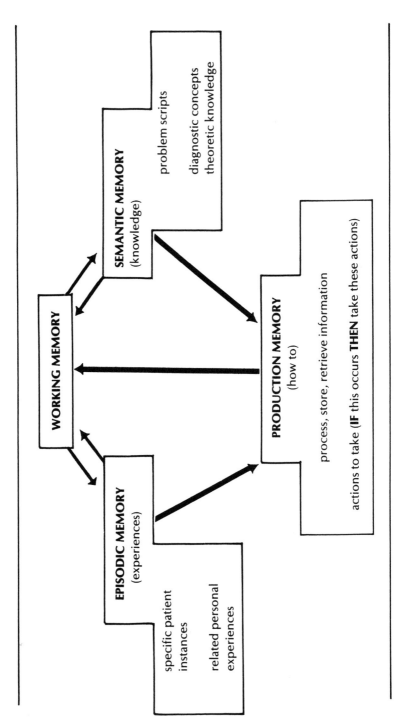

FIGURE 2-3   Relationship of Working Memory to Long Term Memory in Nursing Diagnosis and Treatment Planning

On the other hand, if exposed to the knowledge, nurses will hold in semantic memory a body of nursing knowledge that is generic and relatively similar in structure and process, e.g., the body of knowledge about anxiety; its definition; etiological, contributing, and risk factors; defining characteristics; assessment criteria; principles and rationale for nursing care, and criteria for evaluation. Anxiety associated with specific conditions can also be a part of the body of knowledge. For example: Patrick et al. (1991) list anxiety in 31 conditions or situations in their index; Baker (1991) discusses seven different forms of psychiatric anxiety disorders.

It is wise for nurses to be aware of differences in perceptions and judgments that can occur between nurses or other health care providers arising out of variations in stored events and knowledge. It is also wise to develop one's self-awareness concerning the breadth and depth of personal experience and knowledge of particular situations as these may affect one's level of expertise for diagnosis and treatment planning in a given situation.

Episodic Memory

Episodic memory is the repository for storage of experienced life events. Events and experiences that happened before entry into a professional role obviously are stored in long term memory and can affect professional judgments and decisions. Within the professional experience, episodic memory contains all of the experiences in classrooms and laboratories, in encountering equipment, environments, and clinical documents. Episodic memory includes clinical experiences with patients' situations and responses, families, colleagues, and other components of the health care system. Finally, it can include previous cognitive experiences.

Factors Affecting Episodic Memory

Material from episodic memory is affected by several factors.

Elaborative processing   of experiences in working memory strengthens ease of retrieval (Tulving & Thompson, 1973).

Repetition of experiences   at intervals over an extended period of time tends to make them more retrievable than do experiences massed into a short time block (Baddeley, 1990, p. 156). For example:

Participation in nursing care associated with the labor and delivery experience of several women in a clinical learning block on two successive days would be less well remembered than if those experiences were spread out and repeated over a longer block of time.

Patients' situations and their responses, even within a diagnostic category, will vary widely—few are "typical." Thus, the amount and kinds of personal experience a nurse has with particular patient situations will affect: 1) the range of variability the nurse is prepared to consider in new encounters, and 2) the strength of the memory of past encounters with similar situations (Schmidt, Norman and Boshuizen, 1990).

Recency of experience affects recall. Recent events tend to be more easily recalled. For example[4]:

Several nurses on neurology units participating in a graduate student's research were presented with a case vignette. They were given progressive signs and symptoms of an epidural hematoma. After each progressing cluster of symptoms was described, they were asked to write down their decisions about what action to take. When the exercise had been completed, the researcher gave a presentation on the critical signs and symptoms and the points at which it was crucial to take action in order to prevent further complications. Many of the participants found that they had waited so long to initiate action that the patient probably would have suffered major brain damage. A week later one of the nurses encountered a head-injured patient on her unit who began to exhibit the signs and symptoms discussed in the previous week's case. On the basis of her recent experience with failing to take action soon enough in a simulated case and her memory of the correct actions, she was able to take prompt and correct action.

Distortion is a strong possibility in retrieval of information from episodic memory. In general, broad outlines of events are well recalled; however, errors begin to occur with attempts to retrieve greater detail (Baddeley, 1990, p. 310). In addition, what happens after an event can alter one's memory of it (Loftus and Loftus, 1980). Since diagnosis and treatment planning often depend upon accuracy in recalling detail, this can be important. Distortion can be more of a problem when the number of cases experienced is small, so that retrieved information can be skewed by one or two outstanding situations. Memory of experiences also can be distorted by feedback from others, e.g., one nurse in a positive, secure manner recalls the patient situation differently from others, who then revise their memory of it.

These limitations on accuracy of recall from episodic memory may suggest the need for nurses to process clinical events and information in an organized way into related diagnostic and treatment concepts stored in semantic memory, in addition to retaining the patient instances themselves in episodic memory.

Semantic Memory

Semantic memory is that part of the memory system for permanent knowledge storage. This knowledge is thought to be stored in networks of interrelated areas of

---

[4]Personal communication from Pamela Mitchell, RN, PhD, FAAN, Professor, Physiological Nursing Department, University of Washington. Example used with permission.

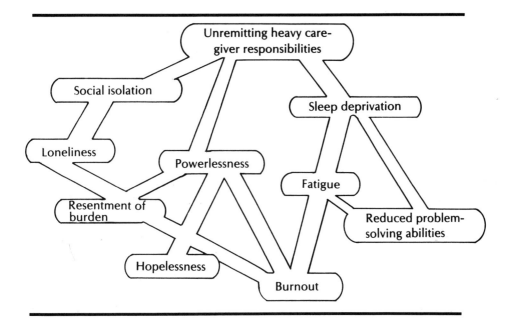

FIGURE 2-4   Example of Linkages Between Diagnostic Concepts in Long Term Semantic Memory

knowledge and concepts as illustrated in Figure 2-4. In clinical judgments and decision making, the cognitive processes are those of gaining access to and retrieving information from these networks. Since diagnosis and treatment planning involve use of diagnostic and treatment concepts, the discussion of semantic memory will use this perspective.

Activation of Memory for Diagnosis

Access to semantic memory is gained by the transmission of a unit or chunk of information from working memory to long term memory. This accessing signal contains one or more characteristics that are **common, frequent, essential** properties of the diagnostic concept. In nursing diagnosis these accessing signals would be the risk factors and major and minor characteristics of a diagnostic category. For example:

A 55-year-old single woman on a disability retirement from her university professorship has had a diagnosis of Parkinson's disease for seven years. She is now dependent upon her widowed older sister, with whom she lives, for much of her care. The sister has brought the patient to the parkinsonism clinic because of the patient's increasing difficulties in eating and her own frustration in dealing with them. The clinic nurse makes a home visit during lunch to observe the patient's eating behavior. She notices that the patient puts too much food on the fork at some times and at others raises an empty fork to the mouth, uses only one hand, seeks food with the fork outside of the plate, spills food en route from plate to mouth, misses the mouth with the fork, chews without food in the mouth, has difficulty in biting off pieces of bread, forces swallowing, stops eating when there are any distractions nearby. She also notices lack of facial mobility.

The accessing signals in this instance are 1) data on the history of advanced Parkinson's disease, 2) the cluster of specific changes in self-feeding behavior and facial immobility.

Accessing long term memory is thought to begin at one concept and then to spread along connecting pathways to intersect with other related concepts. For example:

The accessing chunk in the example above could lead to the diagnostic concept of "feeding self-care deficit" (Carpenito, 1989) and then to Parkinson's disease, or more specifically, advanced Parkinson's disease. Both concepts need to be retrieved in order to fully understand the patient's situation as a basis for planning treatment. The unit of information on lack of facial expression could access to the concept of communication. For the sister the chunks of data related to frustration and lack of knowledge about parkinsonism would be the accessing triggers.

The nurse's diagnostic network might also have pathways that lead to activation of related concepts, such as potential for nutritional deficit, self-concept distur- bance, impaired communication, impaired individual or family coping, and burnout.

The patient manifestations in this situation were fairly typical of the eating difficulties and loss of facial expression experienced by individuals with advanced parkinsonism (Athlin et al., 1989 ; Linde, 1993). The sister's reported frustration and lack of knowledge about helping strategies with the advancing disability are not uncommon.

Typical or prototype information is stored centrally in the concept, while the atypical is more peripheral and therefore slower and more difficult to access. Sim- ilarly, situations involving highly interrelated concepts can be judged more accu- rately and quickly than those with weaker relationships.[5]

Activation of Memory for Treatment Decisions

Treatment decisions logically are made after the specific diagnosis and prognosis have been determined. The information chunks from working memory used to access treatment elements of concepts would include:

- the *specific* nursing diagnosis, and
- the nursing prognosis.

[5]This has implications for storage of knowledge in semantic long term memory and will be discussed later in this chapter and again in Chapter 7.

Given the example above of the woman with Parkinson's disease and the primary caregiver (her sister), the chunks of data in working memory used to access knowledge for treatment would include:

Pt. Dx:
    Progressively impaired eating self-care R/T parkinsonian concentration deficits, impaired muscle coordination, and rigidity.

    Potential for impaired communication R/T parkinsonian facial immobility.

Caregiver Dx:
    Impaired coping with eating problems of pt. R/T knowledge deficit about advanced Parkinson's disease and treatment options L/T frustration and possible burnout.

    Potential for impaired interpretation of patient's feelings, interest, and current intellect R/T loss of facial expression.

Pt. prog:
    Progressive difficulties with eating and other self-care activities. Relationship with sister positive, but lack of facial mobility can hamper communication.

Caregiver prog:
    Capable and desirous of learning about disease and care strategies. Able to implement if she receives support and respite.

Such chunks in working memory can activate knowledge about:

- The range of treatment options available to compensate for the parkinsonian deficits in coordination and concentration at mealtime and the knowledge base that supports them.
- Principles of adult teaching/learning.
- Risks of misunderstood communication with reduced facial expression and strategies of adaptation.
- Changing role relationships from interdependency to dependency.
- Professional, personal, and community resources for gaining long term support and respite.
- Risk factors for burnout and preventive strategies.

Knowledge about treatment options and rationale are stored on pathways closely linked to the diagnoses or situations they are meant to address. And, since some treatments are applicable to more than one diagnosis, treatment knowledge would have a network to permit these linkages, just as there were linkages between related diagnoses in the diagnostic phase.

When the nurse has encountered particular diagnoses or situations many times, the movement from working memory to treatment elements of episodic-semantic memory can become very automatic and rapid. Experts come to have little awareness of their processing of information (Berry and Broadbent, 1984).

Production Memory

One cognitive scientist has theorized that there is a separate form of long term memory discrete from episodic and semantic memory. It is memory concerned with procedures—the "how to's." He has called it "production memory" (Anderson, 1985). The proposed memory linkage is: "**IF** situation A exists **THEN** Action B is taken." For example, **IF** the person is choking on a piece of food, **THEN** do the Heimlich maneuver. In nursing there are some situations when this rapid, automatic IF–THEN memory and action are crucial to patient well-being, but there are also some risks associated with routine and automatic use of an IF–THEN approach. Particular patient situations and responses in the nursing domain have commonalities (or one couldn't diagnose them); however, there can be many variations in both situation and response that should affect both diagnosis and treatment. These require retrieval of a network of possibilities in semantic memory, not automatic responses. The effective nurse learns when an IF–THEN memory approach is appropriate and when it is not. And this too is a part of one's long term memory. See *Exercise Set 2–7.*

The *cognitive* procedures associated with diagnostic thinking and treatment decisions can also be stored in procedural memory.

For exercises on long term memory see *Exercise Set 3.*

Stages in Development of Memory Use in Clinical Practice

Diagnostic and treatment decisions can be made more efficient by systematically storing knowledge so that it can be retrieved when it is needed. It has been theorized that, in acquiring expertise in use of memory for diagnosing and treating health-related problems, individuals go through several stages (Tanner, 1984; Benner, 1984; Schmidt, Norman and Boshuizen, 1990). Development of expertise involves each part of the memory system. The following description of stages in clinical thinking has been adapted from work done by Schmidt, Norman, and Boshuizen (1990) with medical students and physicians. Table 2-1 and the discussion that follows adapts the original medical perspective to that of nursing students and clinicians.

Stage 1. Preclinical

In the preclinical stage, preparation of memory for clinical practice is begun through classroom-oriented experiences. *Sensory memory* is trained to recognize and attend to stimuli coming in from the environment, e.g., feeling a pulse, recognizing systolic and diastolic heart sounds, bowel sounds, the sight of chest excursion in breathing, or changes in color. Preparation of *working memory* involves illustrations

TABLE 2-1 Stages of Development of Memory for Clinical Judgments and Decisions

Stage 1 Pre-Clinical	Stage 2 Early Clinical	Stage 3 Increased Clinical	Stage 4 Advanced Practice
Theoretical foundations taught to begin building diagnostic and treatment concepts and discipline-specific language to encode stimuli.	Beginning encounters with patients and families. Conscious use of theoretical knowledge to explain observed phenomena and situations. Beginning use of discipline-specific language to encode stimuli.	Movement to development of *problem scripts* that use clinical knowledge more than theoretical. Language for encoding stimuli becomes more precise. Continued encounters with patients build a pool of specific instances of various phenomena and situations.	Increasing pool of instances leads to use of *patient instance scripts* to recognize and explain recurring phenomena and situations. Problem scripts are further developed in terms of incorporating greater variability. Problem scripts are used for less familiar situations. Encoding language in familiar situations becomes more integrative and sophisticated. Diagnoses become more complex and integrative.

that group particular features of the patient situation and increase discipline-specific vocabulary for encoding information in working memory. *Long term memory* is provided with basic information about discipline-specific knowledge and language or adaptation and application of knowledge from other disciplines to the nursing field. Diagnostic concepts are taught in ways that show organization of recognition features and link them to the underlying dynamics. Pathways to other related diagnoses to be considered are also illustrated. Typical cases may be offered through patient presentations or simulations, videos, movies or written materials. Questioning and assignments lead the student to link the memory system's different components. The process is fairly conscious, laborious, and often not particularly efficient.

Stage 2. Early Clinical

At this stage nursing students move into clinical situations, actually encountering patients and families, gathering data and engaging in diagnostic and treatment planning activities. As beginning clinicians, they consciously and often painstakingly seek to link information from the clinical setting with explanatory theoretical knowledge from LTM. In the nursing domain these linkages typically involve knowledge of normal age-related structure and physiology, pathophysiology, human responses to health and illness, the nature of the medical treatment, knowledge about environmental factors, psychosocial knowledge, values and so on. In making a diagnosis, the goal is to use knowledge from LTM in order to understand the dynamics of the observed situation or response, the etiology, and the manifestations. Diagnoses tend to be limited in focus—discrete, multiple, and often quite general.

The amount of clinical experience at this point is limited for many nursing students, so there are few comparable patient situations to recall from episodic memory. There is also limited production memory involving processing of information in working memory and retrieving relevant information from episodic and semantic memory.

With increasing exposure to clinical situations, the initial knowledge structure moves to higher levels as more synthesis occurs. More simplified ways of explaining signs and symptoms associated with diagnostic labels begin to emerge. Earlier, initial explanation of the observed situation required extensive retrieval of all the related knowledge. However, in encountering numbers of similar patient situations, the student finds similarities, begins to reinforce and simplify linkages, and develops knowledge packages containing pertinent, clinically usable information.

Stage 3. Increased Clinical Experience

As additional experience with patient situations is gained, the wordy, conscious explanations of causality and underlying mechanisms are gradually organized into **problem scripts** featuring risk factors, dynamics, and manifestations associated with specific patient problems. Language for encoding stimuli becomes more precise. Students gradually add more variability to the typical case and to problem scripts. They also increase the number of diagnostic areas for which they have scripts. Problem scripts will vary with clinicians depending upon differences in their patient experiences. Diagnoses tend to become fewer, more precise, complex, and integrative as the student sees more relationships among data or phenomena (Thomas and Sanger, 1989).

Stage 4. Advanced Practice

Experienced clinicians develop increasing numbers of **patient instance scripts** (PIS). These are memories of specific patient situations. They are increasingly used in familiar situations as a basis for comparison. More sophisticated language is used for encoding experiences. The availability of multiple previous patient experiences in combination with problem scripts becomes the foundation of clinical expertise. Recognition in a new situation comes from recognition or sensing of similarities and differences with past cases. Experts not only have the generic problem scripts of stage 3 but whole files of vivid individual instance scripts that encompass commonalities as well as subtle and wide variations.

Since the nature of clinical practice usually determines the types of patient and family instances nurses can encounter, it can be seen that this basis for diagnostic and treatment expertise can be broad or highly specialized. Nurses' personal, cognitive "libraries" of patient instance scripts for use in diagnosis and treatment decisions may be rich in some areas and almost empty in others. Diagnostic and treatment planning expertise varies within individuals as well as between them.

Building libraries of readily accessible diagnostic packets (problem scripts) and patient instances that will be adequate for expert nursing practice is the goal of every nurse who seeks to become an expert clinician. This valuable collection grows day by day, requiring ongoing attention and effort that any type of valuable collection does.

In this book the reader will find one system for organizing general problem scripts in Chapter 7. In addition, throughout the book there are numerous vignettes providing data that can be placed into patient instance scripts.

For exercises dealing with stages of development of memory for clinical purposes see *Exercise Set 4.*

Summary

Knowledge of the nature of memory and its relationship to clinical judgments and decision making is important. The limitations of sensory and working memory emphasize the importance of developing strategies for effectively managing these limitations. Understanding the potential richness of each component of long term memory can help nurses to value ongoing investment in their memory bank. This means not only making regular, significant deposits of knowledge, experience, and skills, but also developing efficient storage systems for ease of access to these deposits when they are needed.

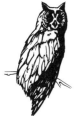

Exercises Related to Understanding and Use of Memory

Set 1 □ Sensory Memory

1. Engage in the following exercise to gain a sense of the encoding of stimuli that occurs in sensory memory.
   Gather or recall five different forms of stimuli from patient situations: a) assign descriptive word(s) to the sensory stimuli you experience, e.g., the sound, the tactile sensation, the smell, the sights; b) assign the professional word that describes the type of data, e.g., radial or pedal pulse, bowel sound, distended neck veins, circumoral pallor.
2. Engage in the following exercise to gain an awareness of how one learns to attend to selected stimuli coming in to sensory memory from the patient situation yet ignore others.
   Find or think of a familiar nursing diagnostic area or patient situation. Think of/list the data that are important to attend to when you next encounter this situation.
   Then think of a nursing diagnostic area or patient situation with which you are not familiar. List the stimuli that you would think important to attend to.
   Compare the two lists and consider the implications for your practice.

Set 2 □ Working Memory

1. From the material developed in Exercise Set 1, seek to further transform/encode the data into mental information that will be helpful in nursing diagnosis. Describe each piece of mental information from sensory memory in as precise professional or nonprofessional language as possible.
2. Recall a clinical judgment you made "without really thinking about it"—one that seemed to happen quite automatically. Ask yourself, "How did I know that?" Notice the patient data you probably processed in your WM to arrive at the judgment you made. If you are not yet having patient experiences, try the same exercise in nonclinical situations.
   Interview a practicing nurse about clinical judgments she or he makes without really thinking about it. Ask the nurse to recall the patient data that enabled her or him to make that judgment.

PATRICK M, WOODS S, CRAVEN R, ROKOSKY J, BRUNO P: *Medical-Surgical Nursing: Pathophysiological Concepts.* 2nd ed. Philadelphia: J.B. Lippincott, 1991.

SALAME P, BADDELEY A: Disruption of short-term memory by unattended speech: Implications for the structure of working memory. *Journal of Verbal Learning and Verbal Behavior* 21:150–164, 1982.

SCHMIDT H, NORMAN G, BOSHUIZEN H: A cognitive perspective on medical expertise: Theory and implications. *Academic Medicine* 65:611–621, 1990.

SQUIRE L, OJEMANN J, MIEZIN F, PETERSEN S, VIDEEN T, RAICHLE M: Activation of the hippocampus in normal humans: A functional anatomical study of memory. *Proceedings of the National Academy of Sciences.* 89:1837–1841, 1992.

TANNER C: Toward development of diagnostic reasoning skills. In Carnevali D, Mitchell P, Woods N, Tanner C (eds): *Diagnostic Reasoning in Nursing.* Philadelphia: J.B. Lippincott, 1984.

THOMAS MD, SANGER E: Diagnostic clusters, holism and reductionism. Paper presented at the Theory and Research-based Psychosocial Nursing Practice Conference. Seattle, WA: University of Washington Psychosocial Nursing Department, July 12–14, 1989.

TULVING E: *Elements of Episodic Memory.* Oxford, Eng.: Clarendon Press, 1983.

TULVING E: Episodic and semantic memory. In Tulving E, Donaldson W (eds): *Organization of Memory.* New York: Academic Press, 1972, pp. 381–403.

TULVING E, THOMPSON D: Encoding specificity and retrieval processes in episodic memory. *Psychological Review* 80:352–373, 1973.

UNDERHILL S: Assessment of cardiac function. In Patrick M, Woods S, Craven R, Rokosky J, Bruno P (eds): *Medical-Surgical Nursing: Pathophysiological Concepts.* 2nd ed. Philadelphia: J.B. Lippincott, 1991, pp. 616–633.

WALDORP M: The workings of working memory. *Science* 237:1564–1567, 1987.

WILD L, CRAVEN R, CUNNINGHAM S: Assessment of vascular function. In Patrick et al.: *Medical-Surgical Nursing: Pathophysiological Concepts.* 2nd ed. Philadelphia: J.B. Lippincott, 1991, pp. 802–811.

3

The Diagnostic Reasoning Process

Diagnostic reasoning is a process that enables an observer to assign meaning and to classify phenomena in clinical situations by integrating observations and critical thinking. This information processing involves sensory, working, and long term memory. It is a series of clinical judgments made during and after data collection, culminating in informal judgments or formal diagnoses. It can be carried out as a deliberate, conscious activity or may occur spontaneously with little awareness.

Times When Diagnostic Reasoning Occurs

Diagnostic reasoning begins as soon as diagnosticians receive information about particular clinical situations in which they will be involved—even before entering the situation or meeting the patient. It continues or recurs throughout the initial assessment and after leaving the patient situation as well as in subsequent encounters.

Diagnoses Are Made When Data Become Available

Often it is not possible to make a sufficiently precise diagnosis in the first patient encounter. One senses the existence of a problem area but sufficient data to make a specific diagnosis are not available. For example:

The patient's physiologic status limits the giving of subjective information.

The patient may not share sensitive and important information during the initial assessment.

Behavioral and physiological responses may become observable only under certain conditions not present during the initial assessment.

The occurrence of a behavior or response in a single situation may be regarded as insignificant until it recurs.

Data on external resources or home environment may not be available.

When these conditions are present, data collection and diagnostic reasoning involving possible problem areas continue as data become available until a valid nursing diagnosis specific enough to guide treatment can be made and other diagnoses can be ruled out.

Nursing Diagnoses Change

Nursing diagnoses tend to be much more dynamic and transitory than medical diagnoses. For example:

The diagnosis of diabetes mellitus tends to be a lifetime medical diagnosis, but the nursing diagnoses associated with patient and family responses to living with the effects of diabetes and its treatment will change many times as daily living, functional capacities, and external resources change.

Even time-limited medical diagnoses, such as normal pregnancy, a sprained ankle, or pneumonia, may be accompanied by nursing diagnoses that change during the time the medical diagnosis is valid.

Therefore, even though initial nursing diagnoses are accurate and precise, they probably will need to be revised several times during the course of nursing care associated with a particular medical diagnosis.

The nursing diagnosis may need to be revised because of changes in:

Patient response or the situation resulting from the effects of nursing treatment: a person with diabetes is taught the skills of self-administration of insulin and self-monitoring and incorporates these activities into daily living.

Patient response in a situation unrelated to nursing treatment: Young parents are caring for a child who is on a ventilator. The father has difficulty tolerating the stress and leaves home. Emotional and physical problems appear for both mother and child.

Daily living in areas affecting the diagnosis: The person who has been undergoing diagnostic activities to determine whether she has cancer or not has been using denial as a means of handling the uncertainty. The tests come back positive, and she faces a conference with the physician in which she will be confronted with the findings and be asked to undergo some aggressive medical treatment.

Patient's environment—placing different requirements on functional capacities: The man who has had a serious myocardial infarction and who is very frightened transfers from the coronary care unit to the telemetry unit where staffing is much less.

External resources affecting the patient's health situation: The car breaks down and public transportation is not usable, a job is lost, an excellent 911 emergency system is available, the local cancer or diabetes associations are very active and supportive.

Whenever there is a change in the patient, the medical treatment, the related daily living, the caregivers, the environment, or external resources, it is probable that nursing diagnoses need to be revised. This involves collection of current data and use of diagnostic reasoning to discontinue or revise present diagnoses or develop new diagnoses that are currently appropriate. Thus, diagnostic reasoning is a continuous behavior in nursing practice. A hallmark of expert nursing practice is the ability and willingness to remain open to changes in the clinical situation.

Nursing Process and Diagnostic Reasoning as a Progression

Nursing process is the approach often used to introduce diagnostic thinking to beginning students. In describing nursing process the first two steps, data collection and data analysis (diagnosis), are pictured as either being separate or only slightly overlapping, as shown in Figure 3-1. This is a highly appropriate approach for beginning clinicians who have limited knowledge in the field, only a beginning command of the requirements of the professional role and role relationships, novice level skills in interviewing and assessment within the framework of a nursing database, and perhaps some initial discomfort in relating to patients and their families. With these limitations, the skills of data collection and analysis are probably most easily learned and more accurately carried out as separate operations.

However, when the clinician develops more theoretical knowledge and clinical experience and is able to be more observant, flexible, and creative in assessment encounters with patients and families, a change in thinking begins to occur (Elstein, Shulman, and Sprafka, 1978; Tanner, Padrick, Westfall, and Putzier, 1987). The

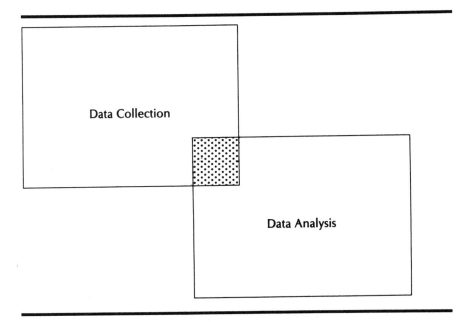

FIGURE 3-1 Overlap of Data Collection and Analysis in First Two Elements of Nursing Process. Adapted from Carpenito L: *Nursing Diagnosis: Application to Clinical Practice,* 4th ed. Philadelphia: J.B. Lippincott, 1991, p. 47

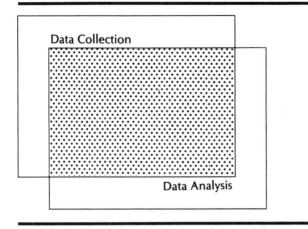

FIGURE 3-2   Overlap of Data Collection and Analysis in Diagnostic Reasoning

two steps of data collection and analysis begin to merge. There is more overlap between them as shown in Figure 3-2. The diagnostician begins to interpret and make judgments about the data as they are received. These judgments, in turn, shape the subsequent data gathering and thinking.

The activities of taking in data, processing the information, and assigning meaning and labels to represent the real clinical situation are the subject of the remainder of this chapter. It is hoped that, with an understanding of the elements of the diagnostic reasoning process, the reader will be able to gain the requisite insight and skill for movement from novice to expert nursing diagnostician.

Elements of the Diagnostic Reasoning Process

One of the ways to understand a complex process that cannot be observed is to illustrate it in a diagram and to describe the elements. Unfortunately, a diagram usually results in an oversimplification of the reality it is supposed to represent. This is certainly true in the complex cognitive activity of diagnostic reasoning. For example, the process described in this chapter will probably seem quite linear as it is diagrammed. It might even seem that one should move straight through the elements as they are diagrammed and described. In practice, the process is much more integrative. For this reason, as you read, notice that both data collection *and analysis* occur in almost every element of the diagnostic reasoning process as indicated by the asterisk in front of the elements in Figure 3-3. Note also that Figure 3-3

Collection of Pre-Encounter Data about Patient Situation*

*Entry into the Patient Situation

    Make a quick overview
    Do an urgency scaling for data collection or action
    Determine strategies for gathering patient data
    Structure role and nursing perspective for patient

*Collection of Data Using Screening or Problem-Oriented Approach

*Coalescing of Data into Related Chunks in Working Memory

*Selection of Cue or Cue Cluster of Highest Priority for Initial Diagnosing

*Retrieval of Possible Diagnostic Explanations or Patient Instances from Long-Term Memory

    Move from general to specific
    Consider competing or alternative diagnostic explanations

*Utilization of Recognition Features Associated with the Retrieved Diagnostic Concepts as Guides for Observation of Patient and Situation

*Comparison of Data in Patient Situation to Recognition Features in Diagnostic Concept, Problem Script, or Patient Instances

*Assignment of a Diagnosis if the data fit the recognition features of one of the retrieved diagnoses, problem scripts, or patient instances.

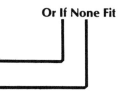

Or If None Fit

---

*Pre-encounter data may or may not involve clinical judgment. If information is deliberately sought out by the nurse, judgment is involved. If the nurse is exposed to data without taking initiative no clinical judgment is involved.

FIGURE 3-3   Components of the Diagnostic Reasoning Process

describes the process in terms of components, *not steps*. Thus, while "diagnosis" is formalized and described as a component at the end of the diagram, the diagnostician will have been retrieving and considering diagnostic possibilities, making diagnostic judgments, and adjusting actions as a part of elements much earlier than this appears in the diagram and descriptions.[1] In fact, accurate diagnosis depends on this suppleness in thinking and adjustment of assessment behavior. Judgments made during data collecting can have a major influence on the diagnosis. Therefore, it is important to know about them—when they occur, how they function, and ways in which they can help or interfere with accurate, precise diagnosis.

The diagram also seems to suggest that diagnosis may be completed in one assessment interaction. Often initial diagnoses can be made with the patient or family member whose problems are quite obvious and clearcut—or with those who are clearly managing effectively the health situation requirements. It is not uncommon, however, for the diagnostic process to be carried out over several encounters with the patient, the family, and with other sources of patient data to identify initial problem areas. Thus, the movement to diagnosis may involve several loops back through earlier elements. Diagramming such integration and movement within the elements would probably make the picture undecipherable. Therefore, consider the diagram in Figure 3-3 to represent elements and relationships that have been found to occur in the diagnostic reasoning process but maintain an awareness that the reality of human behavior in diagnostic reasoning is much more complex.

Collection of Pre-encounter Data About the Patient Situation

One strategy diagnosticians use to keep diagnostic tasks within their working memory's limited capacity is to begin to narrow the field for data collection early. It is done initially by using information about the patient or clinical situation that becomes available even before seeing the patient. This information may be available from several sources:

■ *Word of mouth:* Someone who has had phone contact or personal contact with the patient or situation (remember that such data has already been screened through the reporter's senses, thinking and language, so it has been modified by that person's interpretation and use of language).

---

[1] In research on diagnostic reasoning in both medicine and nursing, it has been found that both students and clinicians begin to consider diagnostic possibilities and make diagnostic judgments *very* early (Neufeld, Norman, Feightner, and Barrows, 1981; Elstein et al., 1978; Kassirer and Gorry, 1978; Benbassat and Cohen, 1982; Tanner, 1981; Putzier, Padrick, Westfall, and Tanner, 1985; Tanner, Padrick, Westfall and Putzier, 1987).

- *Written material:* Admission records, intake records, previous health care records (these also involve interpretation).
- *Generalizations about patients:* Patients who utilize a particular service (e.g., crisis clinics, women's health clinics), ethnic groups, lifestyle, religious affiliations, age groupings, address or lack of a permanent address, fame or notoriety, occupation, status, etc.

Use of Pre-encounter Data

One way in which information received prior to entering a patient situation is used is to direct one's attention. It suggests that some areas of data collection will be extremely important and others can be safely delayed or omitted.

Physicians routinely use pre-encounter information on age and sex as a basis for shaping their assessment. For example:

Prostatic problems are not considered among prepubescent boys or females of any age but are a highly significant area of investigation among men over 60.

Breast neoplasms are not a high priority investigation among prepubescent females or males of any age but are important areas for regular assessment among adult females and particularly elderly females.

Nurses also use pre-encounter information on age and sex as well as other variables. For example:

With infants or children young enough to be fully dependent on others to meet many requirements of daily living, assessment of the parents' or caregivers' status becomes an important focus of attention. With self-sufficient adults it is not an early consideration.

Adult females are more likely to have responsibility for the care of others than are males. Caregiving responsibilities in relationship to functional capacities may be an important avenue for investigation among adult females but may have less priority among adult males.

Nurses use other demographic data in shaping the directions their assessments will take. For example:

Home addresses give a sense of neighborhood (urban, inner city, suburban, rural), transportation issues, socioeconomic environment, safety risks, ethnicity, air and water quality, ease of access to services and technology, distance from family or support networks, etc. An apartment designation suggests certain levels of home responsibility, a nursing home or retirement home another, single dwelling or rural another, and no home address still another.

Name, relationship and address or phone number of "person to notify" identify the available or preferred support system and suggest areas of data needed to determine the nature and level of support that this person or others might provide and also give some idea of geographic distance from identified support person.

Certainly, data from the health care setting itself and knowledge about the experiences and demands the patient may encounter creates a mind-set that can influence the assessment. For example:

In an emergency room, there is a mental set to begin with physiological and psychological responses to crises of patients and those who are sharing their experience.

On inpatient units associated with clinical specialties such as cardiac, respiratory, diabetes, head injury, allergies, the assignment of patients to such particular clinical units tends to shape nurses' mind-set about the directions of nursing assessment.

An outpatient eye surgery clinic dealing primarily with cataract surgery will influence nurses to think about a different data collection approach than will an outpatient women's health care clinic.

At community mental health centers, nurses are ready to look for cues indicating emotional stressors and responses.

Long term stay settings generate a different mind-set to obtain breadth and depth of data than do short term stay settings.

Outpatient care and home care settings predispose nurses to attend also to the patient's daily living environment, the caregivers and external resources.

Nurses also have pre-encounter data on the nature of demands that will be placed on patients and families within the particular health care setting at this time, e.g., particular diagnostic tests or examinations, medical treatment, use of high technology equipment, stressful or painful experiences. Pre-encounter data about commonly occurring demands of the health care setting will influence data collection.

These examples suggest how commonly available pre-encounter data and the environment itself begin to influence the direction of data search and priorities of attention.

At times, pre-encounter data not only determine what one will notice and the importance assigned to particular areas but also a mind-set to interpret data in particular ways. Some types of patients will be seen as having greater credibility than others. Reported symptoms may be given different interpretations depending on pre-encounter knowledge about the person who is reporting the situation (see Chapter 6, p. 152ff).

Advantages of Using Pre-encounter Data

Effective use of pre-encounter data can enable a clinician to begin appropriately narrowing and focusing the data search field as well as preparing the nurse to attend to important cues in the situation. Any initial encounter with a clinical situation is filled with a greater number of cues than the nurse can notice. Using pre-encounter data about the patient and the environment in which the patient and family will receive upcoming health care can reduce cognitive strain and increase both efficiency and effectiveness in observation and information processing.

Risks of Using Pre-encounter Data

Using pre-encounter data as an influence in subsequent data collection does carry some risks. It is not uncommon for patterns in using pre-encounter data to become so established and routine that one can fail to attend to cues that indicate the need for a different approach. For example:

> In some city clinics, nurses expect individuals to present themselves with conditions that are alcohol-related, particularly on nights after social security or welfare checks have been cashed. A mind-set to see disorientation and stupor as alcohol abuse on such "high risk nights" might prevent seeing cues associated with the correct diagnosis of diabetic coma in one individual.

There are many advantages for both diagnostician and patient when pre-encounter data combined with previous experience prepare diagnosticians to function well as soon as they encounter patient situations. The risks are to the patient or family whose situation is *different from the expected pattern*. A mind-set that could cause a nurse to look for certain data and to interpret from one clinical point of view can lead to blind spots, misinterpretation, and misdiagnosis.

Need for Occasional Checking on Personal Use of Pre-encounter Data

Periodically, it is wise to evaluate the ways in which one is using pre-encounter data and other pre-encounter influences. Questions that may be helpful include:

> Which data do I regularly seek out and use before I go in to make an initial patient assessment?

> Are there data that tend to make me feel more comfortable and better prepared to engage in the patient assessment process? For example:

> ■ Oncology nurses may be more comfortable having data on whether patients know their diagnosis and prognosis or not.

- Psychiatric nurses may feel a need for data on previous history of violence.
- Most nurses feel more comfortable and efficient when they know the medical diagnosis and any previous medical treatment.

How am I using these data during the assessment encounter with the patient? Has it led to any "blind spots?" Am I jumping to conclusions without supporting them with valid data?

See *Exercise Set 1* at the end of the chapter for examples of activities one may undertake to develop awareness and skill in use of pre-encounter data and other diagnostic reasoning skills.

Notice that it is possible to be engaging in clinical judgments even before seeing patients and their health situations. Decision making, whether conscious or not, begins during the earliest portions of the assessment process.

Entry Into the Assessment Situation

Both data collection and clinical judgment activities occur very quickly on entry into the assessment situation. For nurses this initial phase is made up of four parts: quick scanning of the patient situation; initial priority setting of data collection or action; decision making about any special strategies needed in data collection; and structuring the role of the patient in the ensuing assessment interaction.

Scanning of the Patient and Situation

The first activity the nurse engages in on encountering the patient in an assessment situation is that of making a quick overview of the situation. The perspective taken will be affected by one's professional background (e.g., experience and clinical specialty), pre-encounter data, and clinical setting. Nurses have been taught or have independently developed approaches to this initial overview. Some do a quick head to toe; some use the ABC (airway–breathing–circulation) approach. A psychiatric nurse may seek to sense the patient's cognitive state, level of anxiety, and potential for violence. A labor and delivery room nurse will look for signs of the woman's physiologic and psychologic responses to being in labor. A nurse caring for preoperative patients (inpatient or outpatient) will scan for manifestations of difficulty in managing the impending surgical procedure and any characteristics that may affect responses during surgery. This represents expertise and depth in selected areas but may also result in neglect of other areas where significant cues exist.

Based on this initial intake of data, which may be purposeful or out of awareness, clinical judgments, *including consideration of possible diagnoses,*[2] are made about the patient's status and the situation.

See *Exercise Set 2* for activities in initial scanning.

Priority Setting or Urgency Scaling

The initial decision about how to proceed results from urgency scaling or priority setting arising from initial scanning of the patient's situation. These clinical judgments (possibly diagnoses) may suggest an immediate need either to gather more data in a particular area or to take action without further data collection. For example:

> If a patient is in some form of extreme physiological difficulty, such as having great difficulty in breathing, hemorrhaging, being in severe pain, retching and vomiting, appearing pale, clammy and in shock, being about to deliver;

> If the patient is in some form of extreme psychological difficulty, such as panic-level anxiety attack, reacting violently toward others;

> If the parent of an infant who is not seriously ill is so distraught as to be creating distress for the child;

the priority will be set to treat the physical or psychological emergency and stabilize the patient and the situation before gathering additional data.

In other instances there may be a need initially to set priorities for the kind of data that is sought. One approach is to use a ten-point *urgency scale* for prioritizing data collection. Assigning "1" means that these data are to be collected immediately or no other data would matter. An example of a "1" would be:

> A situation where there is a question of poisoning or overdose: determining what kind of substance was ingested, how much, how long ago, any signs and symptoms, and any action taken.

Assigning a "10" means that the data would be interesting but would not seriously affect either diagnosis or treatment. Obviously, most data from initial scanning fall somewhere between the urgent 1 and the almost irrelevant 10.

See *Exercise Set 3* for activities in urgency scaling.

Decisions on Strategies for Further Data Collection

A second decision, made during the initial scanning, is that of deciding on the strategies for collecting the nursing data.

---

[2]Note that components of the diagnostic reasoning process discussed later in this chapter, i.e., coalescing of cues, selection of priority cue cluster and consideration of diagnostic possibilities, can already be taking place in the early moments of an encounter.

In some circumstances the nurse will decide that it is necessary to collect objective (observable) data. This decision would be made for example when a patient is unable to speak, is unconscious, is preoccupied with physiological dysfunctions, is not speaking the diagnostician's language, and there is no secondary source of data available.

At other times the decision will be made to collect both objective and subjective[3] data but to collect subjective data in a particular way. For example:

If the nurse had an initial impression of a 3+ level of anxiety in a patient, the approach would be to use short sentences and words. The same approach would be used with a patient having only limited comprehension of English or a person with Down's syndrome.

A patient who has dyspnea would be approached in ways that required only brief responses or yes/no answers to questions.

With young children the language and approach would need to be appropriate to their age and vocabulary.

Teenagers would be approached in ways that were as nonintrusive as possible.

With patients who know their diagnosis of cancer, initial strategies would be associated with listening for the words they use to describe their condition, e.g., growth, problem with my blood, my little problem, lump, lesion, tumor, cancer. This would be done in order to continue to use the patient's or family's choice of words during the assessment.

The nurse's verbal and physical behavior may change during the course of the assessment as more data are taken in. However, initial data collection strategies tend to be based on rather rapid initial clinical judgments.

See *Exercise Set 4* for activities in data collection strategies.

Structuring the Patient's Role in the Assessment Interaction

Many individuals have little idea about the kinds of data a nurse may be seeking from them. This is in contrast to their expectations about sharing data with other health professionals. They know they are going to talk about tooth and gum problems with a dentist and open their mouths for examination. They know they are going to remove their shoes and stockings and talk about foot problems with a podiatrist. They know they will talk about eating and food with a nutritionist. Within the medical profession they have a sense of the kind of information and physical data physicians will seek, in general and by specialty. But few are very clear on what data a nurse would seek. They need to know the kinds of information the nurse will be eliciting in this particular health care situation.

---

[3]Subjective data: personal reports of how the person views the situation, what is being experienced, responses being made, concerns, ideas, and goals.

Most individuals in a patient role, who are able to participate in a nursing assessment, want to feel competent and comfortable in providing data. So the nurse provides the patient with a perspective for participation by saying something like:

"I know you have talked to the doctor(s) about your health problems. As your nurse I'll be working with your doctor(s) in their medical care, but I will also be helping you to manage your living with your health situation and its treatment. I'll be able to give you better care if we could talk for a few minutes about how you have been managing your health situation up to now, any concerns you may have. . . ."

Introduction of the patient's role and perspective in providing data should be tailored to **specifics** of the particular situation that patient and family are facing insofar as the nurse knows it at this point.

See *Exercise Set 5* for activities in structuring the person's perspective and role in assessment activities.

Collection of the Data Base

The third component of the diagnostic reasoning process is the body of the nursing assessment—the collection of the nursing database. Two different approaches are possible. One is the screening or comprehensive database. This tends to follow a predetermined format structured by the guidelines or forms used by the institution or agency (Carpenito, 1989). The second is the focused or problem-oriented approach which tends to be determined by the presenting patient situation (based on clinical judgments or preliminary diagnoses made in the initial scanning and urgency scaling).

The screening or comprehensive approach tends to move from general predetermined areas to the specific. However, even within this structured approach, nurses will begin early in data collection to cluster cues and to sense or recognize problem areas. The problem-oriented approach begins with a focused area, identified by either the patient or the nurse, then branches out to discover its impact on various areas of the patient's (and possibly the family's, spouse's or caregiver's) functioning, daily living and relevant external resources.

Using either of these approaches, the diagnostician accumulates increasing amounts of data. The cognitive processes of coalescing cues into chunks and retrieving and evaluating diagnostic hypotheses (described next) are integral parts of diagnostic reasoning during this data collection.

See *Exercise Set 6* for activities associated with choosing a general or focused approach in assembling a nursing data base.

Coalescing of Cues

Cues entering into working memory, whether consciously noticed or not, tend to coalesce into clusters (chunks) of related materials. For experts these cue clusters or patterns "just appear" (Barrows and Tamblyn, 1980; McGuire, 1985). However, for beginners it tends to result from calculative reasoning. These cue clusters usually have an identifying "tag" or "label," such as respiratory, shock, sleep difficulties, etc.

As noted in Chapter 2, working memory has a limited capacity of 5–9 chunks. What can vary is the number of cues in each chunk.

The capacity to coalesce cues probably is affected by knowledge but even more by clinical experience with comparable phenomena (Schmidt, Norman, and Boshuizen, 1990). Thus, novices may have multiple clusters with fewer cues in each cluster because both knowledge and clinical experience are limited. Expert nurses will tend to coalesce more cues per cluster, incorporate cues that have greater salience to the situation and have insight into relationships between cues (Tanner, 1984; Corcoran, 1986a, 1986b). For example:

> An experienced home care nurse is visiting an older man who has congestive heart failure that has been managed well with medication and a low sodium diet since his last hospitalization 2 months ago. He lives alone in a small apartment, does his own cooking and has help with the shopping and heavier housekeeping from his son who lives in the same town. On this visit the nurse notices that he is moving around less, sits in a straight back chair—not the easy chair, his respirations are rapid and shallow, he stops to breathe in the midst of sentences, he sighs more, he is wearing slippers—not his usual shoes, and his feet and ankles are swollen. He has continued to take his medications but says he "is not feeling so well these days." When she asks if anything different has been going on in his daily living, he says, "Bill's (his son) been sick . . . , wasn't able to get over . . . to take me to the store last week. . . . I've been eating at the fast food restaurant . . . across the street . . . Bill's feeling better now . . . says he'll be over tomorrow to fill up the frig."

> The cluster of cues for this nurse includes the medical diagnosis of congestive heart failure, previous effectiveness of the medications and daily routines, cues of dyspnea and edema and the patient's strategies for accommodating to them, and the cue about eating in a fast food restaurant where the sodium content of the food is likely higher than his usual diet.

> The cue cluster of beginning nursing students could be quite different if they did not yet have theoretical and experiential knowledge of the pathophysiology of congestive failure, effects of the medications, symptoms of fluid retention, linkage between sodium in the diet and fluid retention, and the likelihood of higher sodium content in food in a fast food restaurant. They might develop several cue clusters, e.g., vital signs, edema, changes in speech, rather than the larger clusters that coalesced critical manifestations.

> See Figure 3-4 (pp. 56–57) for illustration of cue clusters of an experienced nurse and that of a beginning student in this case.

The capacity to coalesce salient cues in relevant patterns is crucial to efficient and effective diagnosing.

See *Exercise Set 7* for activities in cue coalescing.

Selecting Pivotal Cue Clusters

Often patients or their families have multiple problems needing nursing diagnosis and treatment, just as there may be more than one medical problem present. However, because of the limits on working memory, it is not possible to develop the database for all problems simultaneously. For this reason, diagnosticians select the cue or cue cluster that seems to have the greatest urgency or importance as a first step, with the understanding that the other problem areas will be subsequently assessed (Elstein, Shulman, and Sprafka, 1978). For example:

> A nurse practitioner may observe that a 60-year-old man has enlarged and stiff but not red and swollen joints in his fingers, and that he has an arrhythmia, shortness of breath and swollen ankles and feet. Undoubtedly, the first attention will go to diagnosing the cluster of symptoms that may be associated with cardiac problems, and then later, attending to the joint problems.

> A nurse is assessing an older woman with advanced cancer who reports that she finds the days and nights very long and lonely. She is growing weaker and more tired; going to the bathroom is increasingly difficult and painful; she is deliberately decreasing her fluid and food intake in order to reduce the number of trips to the bathroom (Carnevali and Reiner, 1990). For the nurse, the first diagnostic priority would be to gather additional data on the problem of fluid/food intake and difficulty in going to the bathroom. Diagnosing the problem areas of boredom and loneliness would be done through subsequent exploration (Carnevali and Reiner, 1990).

Investigating the presenting situation in an orderly fashion is important, so it is logical to begin with the cue cluster suggesting the greatest threat to life or well-being. This is true whether one is using the structured interview guide or a problem-oriented approach. It is equally important to follow up on the less urgent problem areas so that the patient or family situation is as fully diagnosed as is appropriate.

Selection of a cue or cue cluster as the area for investigation triggers the next element in the diagnostic reasoning process—retrieval from long term memory of possible diagnostic explanations for the initial cues.

See *Exercise Set 8* for activities in selecting pivotal cues.

Retrieval of Possible Diagnostic Explanations from Long Term Memory

The selected cue cluster in working memory becomes a signal for retrieval of possible diagnostic explanations from long term memory. These are sometimes

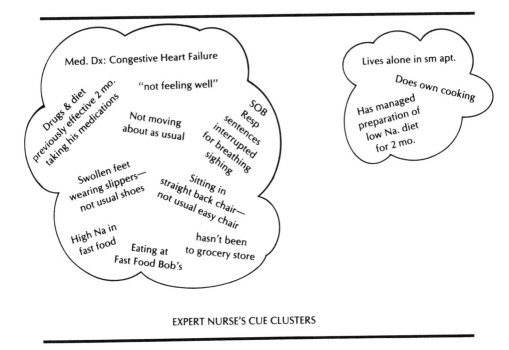

EXPERT NURSE'S CUE CLUSTERS

FIGURE 3-4   Comparison of Expert and Novice Cue Clusters

called diagnostic hypotheses (Elstein, Shulman, and Sprafka, 1978). However, others question whether this use of the word is appropriate (McGuire, 1985, p. 592). Diagnostic explanations may involve utilization of diagnostic concepts, or problem scripts from semantic memory. They may also include patient instance scripts as a basis for comparison.[4] It is important to emphasize the word **possible** since the diagnoses that are initially retrieved may or may not contain the most accurate one. It has been found that the best predictor of diagnostic accuracy is the inclusion of the correct diagnosis within the ones initially considered (perhaps the recognition features are clearer, less disguised or ambiguous) (McGuire, 1985). The strategies for moving toward assignment of a particular diagnostic label to the observed situation involve shifting between recalling the pattern of **recognition features** of the diagnostic concept/problem script/patient instance script and observing the data in the situation. This too can occur with or without awareness.

Two major strategies for arriving at a diagnosis have been described (Elstein, Shulman & Sprafka, 1978). One strategy is to move from a general diagnosis to a more specific one. The second is the development of alternative or competing diagnoses that might explain the observed cues.

[4]See Chapter 2 on memory for discussion of problem scripts and patient instance scripts.

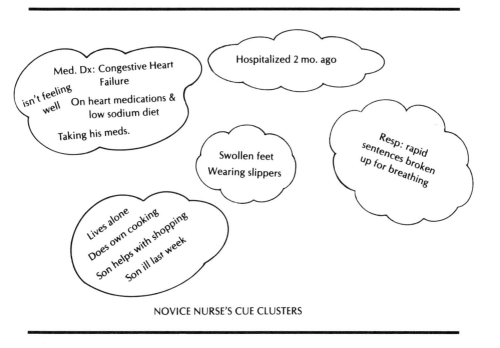

NOVICE NURSE'S CUE CLUSTERS

Movement From General to Specific Diagnoses

This cognitive strategy is a way of limiting the diagnostic task to keep it within the capacity of working memory. First, the general area of explanation is retrieved—for example, the person talks about having sleep difficulties, and the nurse retrieves the general taxonomic category of sleep pattern disturbance (NANDA Taxonomy I Revised, 1990, in Carroll-Johnson, 1991). Then, within this large diagnostic area, more specific diagnoses are considered. These could include:

■ Loss of stage IV (deep) sleep R/T disruptions for child care L/T physical fatigue.
■ Loss of REM (rapid eye movement) sleep R/T ongoing use of sedatives L/T increased irritability.
■ Delayed sleep onset R/T worry about potential homelessness.
■ Fear of going to sleep R/T recurring nightmares (often a pattern in posttrauma syndrome); or for the caregiver, R/T worry over status of the patient.
■ Chronic sleep interruptions R/T such conditions as nocturia, sleep apnea, angina, inadequate symptom management, or caregiving demands.
■ Premature wakening R/T depression/jet lag/time change.
■ Unsatisfying sleep patterns at night R/T napping during the day.
■ Caregiver's chronic sleep deficit R/T patient's sleep apnea, pain, restlessness, terminal status.

It is important to develop hierarchies of diagnostic areas within general categories. The *International Classification of Diseases* is an excellent example of movement from general to specific. General headings include diseases in the categories of neoplasms, infections, trauma, etc. Pages and pages of subsequent headings enable physicians to move to more specific diagnoses and even stages within those diagnoses.

Similarly in nursing, one can move from the general to the specific. The NANDA taxonomy is in the process of further developing these levels in Taxonomy II (Fitzpatrick, 1991). From the existing major NANDA category of *"Exchanging,"* second level category of *"Altered Nutrition"* and third level category of *"Less than Body Needs,"* it is possible to extrapolate more specific categories of diagnostic possibilities. A sample of such extrapolations is shown in Table 3-1. As can be seen, each of these diagnostic possibilities at the more specific levels would have its own antecedent events and risk factors, related factors and major and minor defining characteristics.[5] It is at these more specific levels that it is possible to plan individualized treatment.

How specific should a diagnosis be? Certainly it should be as precise as the observed data permit. Sometimes only a general diagnosis is initially possible because the diagnostician does not yet have enough data to make a more precise one—greater precision must await further data. Ideally, a final nursing diagnosis should be specific enough to permit appropriate therapy. For example:

> Nurses cannot treat nutritional difficulties without knowing the specific nature of those difficulties, their etiology, related factors, and impact on their daily living.

Even within a specific diagnosis, one may need to determine a level of human response. For example:

> Four levels of anxiety have been established, ranging from mild to panic. Learning and problem solving are possible at the lower levels but not at the higher levels. External stimuli in the environment also need to be varied in accordance with the severity of the anxiety. Therefore, a correct diagnosis of anxiety, related factors, and patient response could still result in ineffective treatment if the anxiety level were not specified.

The ultimate aim in moving from general to specific diagnoses is to arrive at a valid diagnosis precise enough to permit effective individualized treatment. This often means creating a more specific diagnosis than a general taxonomic label found on standard plans of care or nursing protocols. Contrast the treatment plan that would be devised with a general diagnosis of:

> "Grieving R/T loss of renal function"

compared with the more specific diagnosis of

> "Grieving (anger depression) R/T loss of preferred lifestyle 2° time demands and dietary restrictions of dialysis."

---

[5]It is interesting that Florence Nightingale, in her 1859 book *Notes on Nursing* in Section XIII "Observations of the Sick," addressed differential diagnosis between appetite and digestion (Seymer, 1954).

TABLE 3-1 An Example of Hierarchical Arrangement of Diagnoses

Exchanging
  Altered nutrition
    Less than body needs
      Agitation and restlessness precluding eating
      Aversion to meat
        Age related
        Resulting from x-ray treatment of GI tract
        Vegetarian preferences
      Depression-related anorexia
        Occurring with adjustment to new diagnosis or recurrence of signs & symptoms
          of life threatening disease
        Grieving
        Organic mental illness
      Forgetting to eat
      Inability to prepare food
        Cooking difficulties
          Lack of: cooking facilities
                   skills
          Impaired physical capacities, vision deficits, neuromuscular deficits, asthenia
        Shopping difficulties
          Lack of: mobility
                   money
                   transportation
                   vision
                   literacy
      Inability to eat
        Chewing difficulties
          Arthritis of jaw
          Dentition status
        Dry mouth
        Dysphagia
          Agnosia, oral
          Apraxia, oral
          Erroneous conditioning
          Pharyngeal paralysis
        Malodorous lesions
        Mucositis
        Sordes
        Structural changes (e.g., head and neck surgery)
      Preference for alcohol over food
      Primary caregiver/food preparer lacks:
        Belief in the necessity of providing for special nutritional needs of patient
        Capability of providing/preparing food
        Interest in patient's nutritional needs
        Understanding of dietary requirements
      Suicidal intent

Adapted from Table 4-1 Exempel på hierarkisk oppbygning av diagnoser. In Carnevali D. *Sykepleieplanlegging.* Oslo: Gyldendal Norsk Forlag, 1992.

Generating Alternative or Competing Diagnoses

It becomes very easy, in the rush of day-to-day practice, to accept the first diagnosis that comes to mind and then to make the data fit the diagnosis rather than make the diagnosis fit the data. It is a bit like forcing a person's foot into the available shoe rather than finding a shoe that will fit the person's foot. Additionally, it is very easy to ignore or explain away nonconfirming data or to ignore the absence of signs and symptoms that should be present if the diagnosis is a valid one. So, in addition to moving from general to specific, it is necessary to consider alternative or competing explanations—differential diagnosis.

The strategy of considering several different but plausible explanations for the same phenomenon or situation is a useful one for guarding against premature closure on diagnostic options. For example:

The nurse sees a cue cluster indicating that the patient or family are not participating in a prescribed treatment regimen or in desirable health behaviors. The initially retrieved diagnostic possibility is that of "Denial stage of adaptation to a diagnosis."

Possible competing diagnoses could be:

■ Conflicting values about the appropriateness, importance, or efficacy of the treatment regimen.
■ Presence of environmental barriers that prevent carrying out the prescribed regimen.
■ Fatigue, asthenia, pain, or other symptoms that prevent participation.
■ Lack of physical coordination, joint flexibility, money, or skills to permit participation in treatment regimen.
■ Priorities in daily living that do not include the activity (e.g., giving care to other individuals).
■ Resistance from others in the support system to carrying out the treatment or health care regimen.

It can be seen in these examples that differential diagnosis is needed in order to provide a more precise diagnosis as a basis for understanding the phenomenon and treating the problem. Just as the specific bacterial or viral agent involved in pneumonia must be diagnosed as a basis for specific medical treatment, so the nursing diagnosis must be precise enough to permit effective treatment. One does not treat "noncompliance," one treats the situation creating the nonparticipation. Nor is there usually one single treatment. Treatments would be different for each of the competing diagnoses above. Thus it becomes crucial to make a differential diagnosis. The first step in making a differential diagnosis is being able to retrieve the diagnostic possibilities from long term memory.

See *Exercise Set 9* for activities in retrieval of diagnostic possibilities.

Content of Diagnostic Concepts

Diagnostic reasoning is enhanced by organizing knowledge about phenomena in a consistent structure. The content and structure of diagnostic concepts/problem scripts, and the associated activities in personal development of one's library of diagnostic concepts are covered in Chapter 7.

When possible diagnoses are retrieved from long term memory, they contain not only the label but other content as well. Of particular importance to diagnostic reasoning are the label, the recognition features or characteristics, and their linkage to the phenomenon. These give the diagnostician:

- A guide for observing or collecting data from the patient situation, a sense of patterns of risk factors and manifestations.
- Language to describe the manifestations.
- An understanding of why these manifestations reflect the presence of the phenomena in this diagnostic category and the linkage between risk factors and the phenomenon or situation.
- Linkages to alternative or competing diagnoses.

Diagnostic labels are important, particularly as they communicate the level of specificity and precision at which the diagnosis is being considered. These labels also eventually tend to represent the reality of the situation for the diagnostician, so it is important that they be accurate and precise.

Recognition features associated with any diagnosis include:

- *Risk factors:* these are elements in the person or the situation that increase the likelihood that this diagnosis will occur. Risk factors can include:

  - Some characteristic of the person being diagnosed, such as age, roles in daily living, self-concept, status of dependency, deficits in particular functional capacities, pathophysiology, altered structure.
  - Environment for daily living (previous/present).
  - Patterns in daily living.
  - Values and beliefs.
  - Status of external resources and support network.
  - Antecedent events—previous health problems, experience with particular diagnostic tests, medical treatments, health care experiences or health care personnel, and health care environments that increase the likelihood of the response associated with this diagnostic category.

- *Manifestations:* these are the patterns of reported or observable findings associated with the diagnosed category. They include critical (major) characteristics that are almost always present if this diagnosis is a valid one and minor characteristics that are frequently associated with the diagnosis. The pattern of manifestations may also include signs and symptoms that *should not* be present if this diagnosis is valid. For example:

- If the observed cues are interpreted to be **anger,** one of the diagnostic possibilities to be retrieved is that of grieving. Two kinds of cues are needed in order to select the diagnosis of "anger stage of grieving." There must be: 1) an antecedent event *experienced as a loss,* and 2) the loss must be of sufficient importance to the person to generate an emotional response. (Table 3-2 illustrates some of the alternative diagnostic explanations for anger and the critical cues that must be present.)

- *Underlying mechanisms:* the underlying mechanisms are those variables and their interaction that create the difficulty or dysfunction and produce a pattern of signs and symptoms associated with the phenomenon. For example:

  - The physiological and behavioral signs and symptoms of acute and chronic pain are different because body systems have adapted to the presence of chronic pain and no longer generate some of the responses that occur when pain is new and acute. Similarly, behavioral responses to the pain change as the individual learns to manage daily living with ongoing pain (Abrams, 1966; Coyle and Foley, 1985; Wheeler, 1993).

For a full discussion of the contents of diagnostic and treatment concepts and the ways of developing them, see Chapter 7.

Use of Retrieved Diagnostic Hypotheses

Patterns of risk factors and manifestations (whether from basic diagnostic concepts, problem scripts, or patient instances) retrieved from long term memory become a **guide** for subsequent observation and data collection (White et al., 1992; Tanner et al., 1987). These patterns structure the diagnostician's ongoing assessment behavior at both conscious and unconscious levels. The presence in working memory of these patterns can shape the next element in the diagnostic reasoning process.

See *Exercise Set 10* for activities in use of recognition features to guide observation.

TABLE 3-2

Competing Diagnoses		Diagnostic Criteria
	Dx (1) grieving— anger stage	Event experienced as a loss + loss of sufficient importance to generate an emotional response
anger	Dx (2) frustration	Significant goal + barrier + strong dissatisfaction
	Dx (3) anxiety	Threat to person + pattern of anger as response to anxiety

---

Comparison of Diagnostic Characteristics With Data in the Patient Situation

The patterns of cues associated with risk factors and manifestations brought into working memory, with or without awareness, are used as a basis for observing cues that are presented and also for collecting more data. The diagnostician is set to notice or actively seeks data that will make it possible to accept, reject or modify diagnostic explanations being considered. At some level of awareness the patient's response or situation is compared with what the diagnostician "knows" about similar situations or phenomena.

See *Exercise Set 11* for activities in comparing recognition features to observed data.

Selecting the Diagnosis or Making the Clinical Judgment

When the characteristics of the diagnosis or clinical explanation fit with data in the patient or situation and when that diagnosis is sufficiently specific to permit treatment, the diagnostician assigns the diagnostic label or accepts the clinical judgment, always with the knowledge that it must remain open to revision or further refinement.

Level of Confidence in the Diagnosis

Diagnostic labels are only inferences about the real situation, so there is clear potential for error. For this reason diagnoses are made with varying degrees of confidence. They may be designated as **impressions, tentative diagnoses,** or **definitive diagnoses.**

Ruling Out Problems

An important element in the diagnostic process is the "ruling out" of problem areas. Ruling out problems requires that the diagnostician match known demands of the health-related situation facing the patient or family with their identified functional capacities and external resources for managing these demands. This means having the data to support one's judgment that the patient or other person(s) have the functional capacities and external resources to manage the present and foreseeable health-related challenges in their daily living. Fortunately, most human beings are able to manage both usual and unusual stresses in their lives. It becomes important as part of the assessment to identify and document areas where patients are managing or can be expected to manage health related challenges without nursing treatment.

See *Exercise Set 12* for activities in ruling out problems.

Validation of the Diagnosis With the Person

Most patients or others closely sharing the patient's health-related experience are able to participate knowingly in the process of identification of their problem areas. When this is true, it is possible to validate one's diagnostic judgments with them. There are, of course, exceptions. For example:

> It probably is not wise to try to validate a diagnosis of "in denial stage of adaptation to new diagnosis" with the person using denial as a current strategy for managing the stress. On the other hand, it may be possible to validate that a patient and spouse prefer to manage the known threat of life-threatening illness by maintaining uncertainty about current status and prognosis.

> Sometimes the nurse is aware of challenges the patient, caregiver, or family will face and the adaptations and skills they will need to undertake, and diagnoses major upcoming difficulties. At this point, it may only add to the person's stress to be presented with such diagnoses.

> The person may not have the insight to understand the situation and may need some treatment before being able to participate in validating the diagnosis.

One area for nursing judgment, then, is when and how to validate initial diagnoses.

The language used in written nursing diagnoses (and medical diagnoses) is highly stylized. It is professional jargon. Thus, in validating a diagnosis with persons being diagnosed, one translates the diagnosis into their language. For example:

> "From what you've told me, I understand that you're really uneasy about your ability to care for your baby when you get home—specifically bathing and caring for the cord and the circumcision. You're also worried about whether he will stop breathing at night the way your sister's baby did 3 months ago. Have I got it right?"

> The diagnosis might be written as: Fear of inability to care for newborn son R/T inexperience and recent SIDS death in family.

Whenever possible, the diagnosis should be shared in a way that will be helpful and will permit that person to validate or contribute to its modification.

See *Exercise Set 13* for activities in validating diagnoses with the person.

Diagnostic Errors

Anyone who engages in diagnostic reasoning can make diagnostic errors. A variety of factors contribute to these errors. Some of these include:

- Equating the ease of remembering specific cases with the probability that they will occur.
- Equating resemblance between specific cases with the probability that they are the same even though some data are missing.

- Expecting certain problems to be present because of frequency of occurrence, the setting, or the time.
- Having so much confidence in one's own diagnostic judgment (even though it may be biased), that areas of data or misinterpretation are blocked out.
- Uneasiness or guilt at having missed a diagnosis in an earlier case and later assigning greater likelihood of its occurrence in order to avoid missing it again.
- Having a value-biased perspective that tends to make one avoid an undesirable diagnosis that is actually present (Dawson and Arkes, 1987).

There are four types of diagnostic errors:

1. Failing to make a diagnosis when there are cues available to indicate that the phenomenon is present and could be diagnosed (**omission of a diagnosis**).
2. Making a diagnosis when cues are present that do not fit with the characteristics of that diagnosis (**making an incorrect diagnosis**).
3. Making a general diagnosis when data are available to permit a more specific, precise diagnosis (**too general a diagnosis**).
4. Making a specific diagnosis, presuming that data not presently available must certainly be present (**making a diagnosis that is unsupported by the data**) (Voytovich and Rippey, 1985).

It is wise to be aware of the potential for errors in diagnosing, whether one consciously acknowledges and verbalizes the diagnosis or makes it without awareness. *Nursing diagnoses are not harmless.* Diagnostic errors can result in inappropriate, ineffective or even harmful treatment in nursing as surely as they can in medicine.

See *Exercise Set 14* for activities associated with diagnostic errors.

Strategies When Initial Diagnostic Hypotheses Do Not Fit the Situation

When risk factors and manifestations are clear-cut and obvious, it is probable that initially retrieved diagnostic hypotheses will contain a correct one. However, patient situations are often much more ambiguous, complex, and elusive. It is not unusual for a nurse to discover that none of the original diagnostic explanations truly fit and lend a solid foundation for effective nursing treatment. When this happens, there are two major strategies to continue the diagnostic process.

Gather More Data

One of the strategies clinicians use when initial diagnoses do not prove adequate is to return to the step of gathering more data. This data gathering can be within the same areas in which data were originally collected or may branch out into other areas that may be linked to the problem but were not touched on in earlier data collection. For example:

The patient has provided data that she knows about her disease and the need to engage in certain activities to prevent further deterioration and maintain her present level of health. Data on her health care practices indicate that she is neglecting these activities in her daily living. The diagnosis of "noncompliance in incorporating prescribed treatment into daily living" is not incorrect but does not lend itself to effective treatment. Competing diagnoses would guide the gathering of data in the following areas:

- Role responsibilities that might interfere with self-care or give priority to other responsibilities.
- Preferences in daily living that conflict with the prescribed regimen.
- Environmental barriers.
- Inability to translate knowledge to actual application in daily living.
- Belief in the efficacy of the treatment.
- Other beliefs about cure and support outside of the prescribed regimen, etc.

Other data gathering approaches include returning to a further review of functional capacities and related daily living requirements or consultation with secondary sources for validation, expansion or modification of earlier data.

Retrieval of Other Diagnostic Explanations

A second strategy is to consider other diagnoses as explanations for the phenomenon or situation being seen. For example:

In Table 3-1 a variety of diagnostic possibilities were listed for the phenomenon of nutritional intake that is less than body requirements. Initially the diagnostician may have chosen 2 or 3 of these that were later unsupported by the data. The subsequent data collection may suggest other possibilities that would be more accurate and specific.

Despite the stress and hurry of the clinical situation, responsibility for diagnostic accuracy and validity requires the nurse to seek a diagnosis that truly fits and explains the presence and absence of data in the patient situation. Nursing treatment is based on it. Patient and family well-being ultimately depend upon it.

See *Exercise Set 15* for activities in use of strategies when initial diagnoses don't explain the situation.

Summary

Diagnostic reasoning is a crucial, ever-present element of professional nursing practice. It is carried out in some fashion whenever a nurse encounters a patient situation, with or without awareness, and whether a diagnosis is put into words or not. Nursing judgments are made and nursing actions are taken or not taken based on both unconscious and conscious judgments and diagnoses. Patients and their families pay for professional nursing services in the belief that actions taken by nurses will be to their benefit and will result in promotion of their well-being and effectiveness in managing health-related daily living. The only way for that to occur is for nurses to be as expert, skillful, and disciplined as possible in the processes they use to make clinical judgments and arrive at nursing diagnoses.

Expertise in diagnostic reasoning is gained slowly. Furthermore, one does not have the same level of expertise in all clinical areas or presenting situations. One can be highly expert in nursing diagnosis in one clinical field or with certain phenomena and relatively ineffective in others. Such awareness is important, since it suggests the need to consult with others in areas where diagnostic expertise is not highly developed. It also indicates that gaining diagnostic expertise is a lifelong pursuit—there is always room to grow.

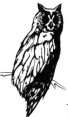

Exercises in Diagnostic Reasoning[6]

Set 1 □ Utilization of Pre-encounter Information

1. Examine completed admission or intake sheets on several patients. Look at:
   A. Name, sex, age, marital status.
   What questions do each of these raise in terms of that patient's and the family's capacities to manage health-related issues? Compare differences between the written information on the patients and consider how this would affect your mind-set for each patient and family if you were to go on to do a nursing assessment for each of them.
   B. Addresses of patient (local, home) and of person to be contacted.
   Is the local address and home address the same? If not, how distant is the home address? What implications does this have for support systems for the patient and knowledge about the resources in the local community? Is the address of the contact person local or distant?
Given the home address, think about the implications this might have for managing health-related problems and data to be collected that arise from the locality and type of housing where the person lives.
   C. Religious designation.
   Are there any particular values, beliefs, or restrictions associated with a designated religious affiliation that could affect patient/family participation in health care in the present situation? If you know the medical diagnosis and

---

[6]These exercises are not "one-timers," but should be undertaken repeatedly in order to gain perspective on the variety and commonalities in clinical situations as well as to gain skill and speed.

potential treatment, are there any that would have priority? Is there potential for cultural beliefs, not designated as "religion," that may be important to know? How could religious and cultural beliefs be explored in data collection (initially, later)?

    D. Physician.

    What do you know about the designated physician's style of practice that may influence data you collect from this patient? For example:

        Some physicians are known to provide information that might be threatening to the patient only if the patient asks directly. Will nursing data be needed on:

            Whether the patient expects to be told without having to ask? Whether he or she will have enough knowledge about the health situation to be able to ask the questions needed? Whether the patient is shy or has language difficulties? (Carnevali and Reiner, 1990, pp. 75–81).

        Other physicians act on their belief that the patient and family need full information about their health situation in order to manage it as effectively as possible. Will you need data on how the patient and family deal with uncertainty? (Mishel, 1988; 1990).

2. Make a list of the kinds of information about a patient and family that tend to make you most comfortable and feeling most prepared to engage in an initial nursing assessment.

    A. Ask yourself why you want each piece of information on your list. Identify specific ways in which your thinking and data collection could be influenced by this pre-encounter data. Are there any data that you prefer not to have before seeing the patient? Why?

    B. Ask expert nurses, fellow students, or nursing colleagues in different clinical settings what kinds of information about the patient and patient situation they really prefer to have before making an initial nursing assessment. Ask how this pre-encounter information affects their approach in the nursing assessment.

    C. Compare different nurses' expressed desire for pre-encounter information with others and with your own. Consider the way in which differences in assessment occur because of pre-encounter data. Identify the advantages. Identify the risks.

3. Choose a patient on whom you are going to make a nursing assessment. Notice the pre-encounter information you have, seek, or receive about the patient and situation. Engage in your usual patient assessment. Afterwards, think back to see if you can determine whether you used any of the pre-encounter information and what influence it had on your assessment approaches and your interpretation of the patient data.

Set 2 □ Initial Scanning

1. Upon entering a patient situation, notice the strategies you use to gain a quick grasp of the situation. What do you look for first? What else do you notice

immediately? Are there any particular environmental features that you notice at this point? If one or more individuals accompany or are with the patient, what do you look for or notice about them?

2. Repeat this activity in several other initial assessment encounters. Do you see a pattern in your scanning strategies? Repeat the exercise in 6 and 12 months. Have any changes occurred? What are they? Why do you think they have occurred?

3. Ask other nurses or nursing students what they notice in their initial scanning of a patient situation. Try to sample nurses or students working in different clinical settings or with patients and families having different health problems. Compare similarities and differences. Do any of their patterns suggest changes that you wish to make in your own? Why?

Set 3 □ Urgency Scaling

1. After completing a nursing assessment, think back to the initial scanning data you noticed. See if you can assign urgency scaling numbers to cues or cue clusters (e.g., 1 = urgent, crucial, needed immediately, to 10 = no hurry, unimportant, might use—create your own criteria for numbers in between). Justify the numbers you have assigned. Do you need a 10-point scale or would a smaller range be as effective?

2. Repeat the activity with different patients.

3. Share your data with your colleagues and with nursing experts. Would they score the data in the same way?

Set 4 □ Decision Making About Data Gathering Strategies

1. After engaging in an assessment interaction, think back to the early stages of it. What cues did you pick up that influenced your subsequent strategies in data gathering? Consider the person's vocabulary, language, hearing status, mental status, awareness of diagnosis, physiological stability, level of consciousness, age, breathing difficulties, other symptoms, speaking difficulties, etc.

2. In what specific ways did these data lead you to modify your assessment behavior? Identify specifically the alterations in your behavior and activities.

3. Repeat the exercise. Each time look for differences in the cues and identify how you modified your data-collecting behavior based on these cues.

Set 5 □ Structuring the Person's Perspective and Role in the Nursing Assessment Interaction

1. Experiment in your thinking with several approaches for providing structure to a person's expectations and actions in participating in the nursing assessment interaction. Talk into a tape recorder and listen to yourself—the content, your language, your voice. Try a variety of versions directed to different patient situations.

2. Role-play the process with partners (nursing students, nurses, non-nurses). Ask them to assume different identities, e.g., a 5-year-old child, a 16-year-old boy, a

suspicious transient, a person with Down's syndrome, a frightened parent in the emergency room whose child has been in an accident, an 80-year-old woman having a cataract removed, etc. After you have described the nursing perspective and their part in the assessment interaction, ask your partners to tell you how they would see themselves *actually participating,* based on the role they have assumed and your presentation. Ask them to identify specifically what you did (words used, voice, body language, actions) that made them feel: 1) more positive and confident about participating . . . more comfortable . . . ; 2) more uncertain . . . less confident . . . uncomfortable.

3. Observe how your patients or other persons participate in the nursing assessments after you have provided your guidelines. Ask your watchbird to notice the words you used, your voice, your body language.

Set 6 □ Choosing a Comprehensive or Focused Nursing Data Base

1. Identify patient situations on your unit, in your institution, or agency in which:
   A. a comprehensive nursing data base is essential/cost effective
   B. a focused nursing data base is more appropriate/cost effective.
   Give the rationale for your decisions in terms of usability of data, time available for collecting the data, and how nursing care would be affected.
2. Select a patient on whom you decide a focused or problem oriented data collection is the approach of choice. Identify the factors that determine what categories of data you collect. Discuss it with a colleague, with a mentor or teacher. Repeat the exercise with other categories of patients.
3. Role play a comprehensive/pre-structured data collection interaction (e.g., a patient with advancing Parkinson's disease or dementia in a home situation, a patient who will have repeated admissions on an oncology unit, a person on a rehabilitation unit, a dialysis outpatient setting). During or after the activity, notice when and how you began to consider possible nursing diagnoses and to gather related data to enable you to make these judgments—even as you followed the structure of the nursing assessment form. Repeat, using an actual patient interaction.
4. Role-play a focused data gathering based on:
   A. a time-limited nursing contact (e.g., an outpatient cataract removal and lens implant, a young woman with 2 children aged 18 months and 3 years and a sprained right ankle and who has come into your hectically busy emergency room).
   B. a highly focused area for current nursing responsibility, e.g., an admission for preoperative care on the morning of surgery, a woman in a mammography clinic, an immunization clinic for children, postoperative care for a patient with a transurethral prostatic resection, a laparoscopic cholecystectomy, a herniorrhaphy.
   Notice how you use the presenting health care problem and treatment to guide the way you approach data gathering about specific areas in daily living that will

be affected by the changed functioning or will require new skills or approaches. Notice how you branch out from the initial narrow focus to gather data on areas where difficulties in patient management are common and nursing diagnoses and treatment often needed. Repeat using an actual patient interaction.

Set 7 □ Coalescing of Cues

1. After completing a nursing assessment with a person, think back to the cues or impressions you received. If possible, try to recall the point in the interaction when you began to "put cues together." Write the cues down, putting them into the clusters that seem to belong together. Did you have labels for the clusters? Repeat the process with several different assessments. Save/file the papers. Repeat the exercise in 6 and 12 months. Contrast the results. Are you putting more cues into each cluster? Are you relating cues that seemed unrelated earlier? Are your "labels" changing? In what way?
2. As you are reading and learning about nursing phenomena, think about the way in which cues cluster into patterns. Think about how they would appear in different patients or individuals.
3. As you listen to other nursing students or nurses report on patients, notice the ways in which they cluster or fail to cluster cues. Think about how you would do it differently or similarly. Give a rationale for your decisions.

Set 8 □ Selecting Pivotal Cue Clusters

1. Using a standard nursing history form for the particular clinical unit on which you are located, gather data according to its structure. As you are moving along, notice if there are any areas where you sense a problem that seems to have greatest immediacy or importance. What cues enabled you to: 1) **sense** the existence of this possible problem area; 2) **assign** it first priority for further investigation.
2. Using a focused/problem-oriented approach to assessment, identify the cues that enabled you to: 1) **sense** the presence of a nursing problem; 2) **assign** it first priority in terms of further investigation. How early in the data gathering did you find yourself beginning to prioritize cue clusters?
3. Periodically repeat these exercises to maintain an awareness of your prioritization of problems. Do you fall into a pattern where you select the same priorities every time for patients with the same types of pathology or medical treatment? Are there other variables causing you to assign the same priorities? Are these valid? Do you think the priorities you are assigning are ones the patient or other person would assign first priority? Under what circumstances would the patient's priority cause you to alter prioritization?

Set 9 □ Retrieval of Diagnostic Possibilities

1. After an assessment interaction, identify the first diagnostic possibilities you considered. How many were there? Did you first identify a general problem

area? Did you move to more specific diagnostic areas? What were they? What competing/alternative diagnostic explanations did you initially retrieve from long term memory? Were there patient instances that came to mind?

Set 10 □ *Use of Recognition Features To Guide Observation*

1. Using the diagnoses you actually retrieved during a nursing assessment, identify the associated defining characteristics that guided your subsequent observation. Include risk factors or antecedent events and manifestations. Write these down and save them. Repeat the exercise in 6 and 12 months and compare your findings. Have they become sharper—more discriminating? How has your exposure to additional theory changed the recognition features you used? How has your added clinical practice modified or reinforced them? Is your vocabulary sharper—more precise quantitatively and qualitatively? Have you encountered more patients who share this same health problem but who are responding differently, so that you are prepared to see greater variability?

Set 11 □ *Comparison of Recognition Features To Observed Data*

1. After engaging in a nursing assessment of a patient or other individual associated with a patient's situation, set up two columns—one for the recognition features of each of the diagnostic possibilities you considered and one for the actual patient data you observed. In the recognition column be sure to note the findings that should be absent as well as those that must be present in order for the diagnosis to be a valid one. In the data column, be sure to include the *incongruent* data as well as data matching the recognition features. Was there a "good fit" between one diagnosis and the data? Did you use your recall of patient instances as a basis for comparison? How?

Set 12 □ *Ruling Out Problems*

1. After an assessment interaction, identify the health-related challenges in daily living (inside or outside the institution) that the patient/family/caregivers/partners are currently facing or are likely to face. Against these challenges, compare the data you obtained on functional capacities, patterns in daily living, values, environment and external resources. Identify the challenges suggested by your data that the patient and those who share the health situation will manage without nursing intervention.
2. Consider your values and what you see as effective management of the health-related situation. Compare this with your data suggesting that the patient/support group will decide they are able or wish to manage without nursing intervention. Is there a likelihood of conflict? If yes, identify.

Set 13 □ *Validating Diagnoses With the Person*

1. As you engage in assessments with several different patients or family members, consider which factors in each situation caused you to decide not to validate a

particular diagnostic area with each one. Discuss the case and your decisions with others to see the range of opinions.

2. Role-play a variety of different approaches you could use in validating a diagnosis, using a colleague or a layperson who is to be the patient, family member, caregiver, or sexual partner. Repeat the experience, varying the age and situation as in the data gathering strategy exercises. Contrast your formal nursing diagnosis with the informal explanatory diagnosis you shared.

3. Consider a variety of different nursing diagnostic areas and experiment with different approaches and language you might use to validate or modify your diagnoses.

4. How do you modify your validation strategies between persons who are overt and confident in their behavior and those who are uncertain and shy and might be fearful of disagreeing; who are distant, reluctant to share data and somewhat suspicious of you?

5. Rehearse the approaches you would use with a person who was adapting to his or her situation by maintaining uncertainty.

Set 14 □ Diagnostic Errors

1. Using your own paper (not the legal patient record), write down your nursing diagnoses for a patient, family member, or caregiver, based on your initial assessment. Set it aside. As the situation unfolds, go back and critique your diagnoses. Were they accurate? Did you miss any diagnoses where findings were available initially but you failed to recognize them or interpret them correctly? Were there data present initially that should have permitted you to make a more specific diagnosis? Did you make any diagnoses based on data that you assumed would emerge but never did? Repeat this exercise periodically to self-monitor your diagnostic performance.

Set 15 □ Strategies When Initial Diagnoses Don't Explain the Situation

1. Recall situations when your initial diagnoses did not fit or adequately explain your findings. What did you do? Did you go back and seek to collect more data before considering any new diagnostic hypotheses? Did you first try to retrieve additional competing diagnostic explanations for the existing data? Which strategies seemed to serve you best?

References

ABRAMS RD: The patient with cancer: his changing pattern of communication. *New England Journal of Medicine* 274:317, 1966.

BARROWS H, TAMBLYN R: *Problem Based Learning: An Approach to Medical Education.* New York: Springer, 1980.

BENBASSAT J, COHEN R: Clinical instruction and cognitive development of medical students. *Lancet* 95–97, January 9, 1982.

CARNEVALI D: *Sykepleieplanlegging*. Oslo: Gyldendal Norsk Forlag, 1992.

CARNEVALI D, REINER A: *The Cancer Experience: Nursing Diagnosis and Management*. Philadelphia: J.B. Lippincott, 1990.

CARPENITO L: *Nursing Diagnosis: Application to Clinical Practice*. 4th ed. Philadelphia: J.B. Lippincott, 1991.

CARROLL-JOHNSON R. (ed.): *Classification of Nursing Diagnoses*. Proceedings of the ninth conference. North American Nursing Diagnosis Association. Philadelphia: J.B. Lippincott, 1991.

CORCORAN S: Task complexity and nursing expertise as factors on decision making. *Nursing Research* 35:107–112, 1986(a).

CORCORAN S: Expert and novice nurses' use of knowledge to plan for pam control: How clinicians make their decisions. *American Journal of Hospice Care* 3(6):37–41, 1986(b).

COYLE N, FOLEY K: Pain in patients with cancer. *Seminars in Oncology Nursing* 1:93, 1985.

DAWSON N, ARKES H: Systematic errors in medical decision making. *Journal of General Internal Medicine* 2:183–187, 1987.

ELSTEIN A, SHULMAN L, SPRAFKA S: *Medical Problem Solving: An Analysis of Clinical Reasoning*. Cambridge, MA: Harvard University, 1978.

FITZPATRICK J: Taxonomy II: Definitions and development. In Carroll-Johnson RM (ed): *Classification of Nursing Diagnoses: Proceedings of the Ninth Conference*. Philadelphia: J.B. Lippincott, 1991.

International Classification of Disease. 9th revision, Clinical Revision 2nd ed. Washington, D.C.: US Department of Health and Human Services, 1980.

KASSIRER J, GORRY G: Clinical problem solving: A behavioral analysis. *Annals of Internal Medicine* 89:245–255, 1978.

McGUIRE C: Medical problem-solving: A critique of the literature. *Journal of Medical Education* 60:587–595, 1985.

MISHEL M: Reconceptualization of the uncertainty in illness theory. *Image: Journal of Nursing Scholarship* 22(4):256–262, 1990.

MISHEL M: Uncertainty in illness. *Image: Journal of Nursing Scholarship* 20:225, 1988.

NEUFELD V, NORMAN G, FEIGHTNER J, BARROWS H: Clinical problem-solving by medical students: A cross-sectional and longitudinal analysis. *Medical Education* 15:315–322, 1981.

PUTZIER D, PADRICK K, WESTFALL U, TANNER C: Diagnostic reasoning in critical-care nursing. *Heart and Lung: The Journal of Critical Care* 14:430–437, 1985.

SCHMIDT H, NORMAN G, BOSHUIZEN H: A cognitive perspective on medical expertise: Theory and implications. *Academic Medicine* 65:611–621, 1990.

SEYMER L: *Selected Writings of Florence Nightingale*. New York: The Macmillan Co., 1954.

TANNER C: Instruction in the diagnostic process: an experimental study. In Kim MJ, Moritz D (eds): *Classification of Nursing Diagnoses: Proceedings of the Third and Fourth National Conferences*. New York: McGraw-Hill, 1981, pp 145–152.

TANNER C: Factors influencing the diagnostic process. Diagnostic problem solving. In Carnevali D, Mitchell P, Woods N, Tanner C (eds.): *Diagnostic Reasoning in Nursing*. Philadelphia: J.B. Lippincott, 1984.

TANNER C, PADRICK K, WESTFALL U, PUTZIER D: Diagnostic reasoning strategies of nurses and nursing students. *Nursing Research* 36(3):358–363, 1987.

VOYTOVICH A, RIPPEY R: Premature conclusions in diagnostic reasoning. *Journal of Medical Education* 60(4):302–307, 1985.

WHEELER VS: Cancer. In Carnevali D, Patrick M (eds): *Nursing Management for the Elderly.* 3rd ed. Philadelphia: J.B. Lippincott, 1993.

WHITE JE, NATIVIO DG, KOBERT SN, ENGBERG SJ: Content and process in clinical decision making. *Image: Journal of Nursing Scholarship* 24(2):153–158, 1992.

4

*Prognostic Judgments in
the Nursing Domain*

Nurses are familiar with the concept of prognosis when it is applied to pathology, pathophysiology and psychopathology. They know that certain pathology can be prevented and that some is cured, either by the body itself or by medical treatment. Other pathology can be stabilized but not cured, while still others progress to death despite treatment. Nurses regularly see that medical treatment decisions are made on the basis of both diagnosis and prognosis. Pathology that can be prevented or cured is treated in one way; that which does not respond to treatment is managed in other ways. Prognostic judgments precede treatment decisions.

Prognosis is less frequently recognized and used as it applies to situations in the nursing domain, and there is at this time little if any research about prognosis in nursing phenomena or about prognostic variables. But nurses in their clinical experience do become aware of the reality that there are varying courses of events and outcomes in human responses to the illness experience, in management of associated daily living, and in availability and use of external resources. They have found that some of these can be prevented or resolved by appropriate nursing treatment and others cannot.

Prognosis is a crucial consideration for nurses in determining nursing goals, treatments, and evaluation. As in the medical field, nursing prognosis is linked to each specific diagnosis.

Modifications in Nursing Process to Incorporate Nursing Prognosis

When nursing prognosis is incorporated into the nursing process, it creates an additional component as illustrated in Figure 4-1. As shown in the figure and as it is discussed in the chapter, prognostic judgments have a major influence on other elements in the nursing process, particularly treatment and evaluation.

The following examples of nursing diagnoses associated with swallowing difficulties illustrate differences in nursing prognoses associated with the dysfunction of painful swallowing.

Dx: Eating difficulties R/T posttonsillectomy pain.
Prog: Resolution of swallowing difficulties and discomfort in 1–2 weeks. Minimal impact on nutritional status.

Dx: Severe eating difficulties R/T esophageal swelling & inadequate pain control 2° radiation esophagitis L/T inability to ingest sufficient calories and continuing weight loss.
Prog: Pain and swelling contributing to eating difficulties will continue for the remaining 6 weeks of treatment and for several weeks thereafter

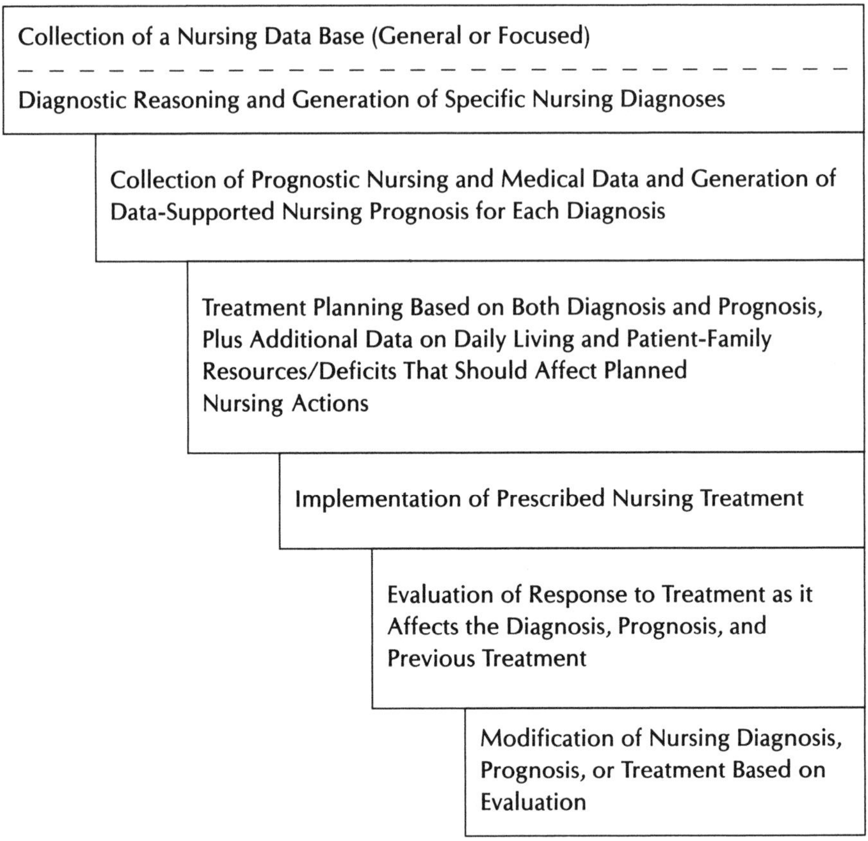

Collection of a Nursing Data Base (General or Focused)

Diagnostic Reasoning and Generation of Specific Nursing Diagnoses

Collection of Prognostic Nursing and Medical Data and Generation of Data-Supported Nursing Prognosis for Each Diagnosis

Treatment Planning Based on Both Diagnosis and Prognosis, Plus Additional Data on Daily Living and Patient-Family Resources/Deficits That Should Affect Planned Nursing Actions

Implementation of Prescribed Nursing Treatment

Evaluation of Response to Treatment as it Affects the Diagnosis, Prognosis, and Previous Treatment

Modification of Nursing Diagnosis, Prognosis, or Treatment Based on Evaluation

FIGURE 4-1   Nursing Process as It Incorporates Nursing Prognosis

with nutritional status threatened. Pain control can be improved and may improve caloric intake.

It can be seen that treatment for each of these examples is quite different and that evaluation criteria and timing for evaluation of response to nursing treatment are strongly affected by both diagnosis and prognosis.

What is Prognosis?

Prognosis is a prediction of the possible or probable course of events and outcomes associated with a particular health status or situation under various circumstances, treatment options or lack of treatment. Prognosis contains several components discussed in more detail in the following pages. The components of prognosis include:

- Areas where changes can occur.
- Types of outcomes.
- Trajectory of change.

Prognostic judgments are based on **prognostic variables,** including dynamics of the diagnosed phenomenon and factors that can affect outcome and trajectory. Data on these variables in the patient's situation are used to predict what the outcome and trajectory will be.

Areas Where Changes May Occur

In the medical domain, areas for change occur in human responses to pathology, pathophysiology, or psychopathology being observed or treated. By contrast, in nursing, the areas where change can occur will include:

- Human responses or functional capacities involved in managing health-related experiences and demands of daily living.
- Aspects of daily living that create health risks or place specific requirements on the patient's or family's functional capacities and external resources.
- Elements of the environment for daily living as they affect health or the presenting problem.
- Availability and capacity to obtain, use, and maintain external resources.

In considering areas for change in a prognosis, it is wise to be specific about the area or areas anticipated to be involved in the prognosis. Specific, rather than general, human responses and associated aspects of daily living, environment, or external resources are involved. For example:

> An older man and his wife had a very active social life prior to his stroke. Many of the activities revolved around eating in social groups. A major residual deficit of his stroke is a form of dysphagia that does not lend itself to rehabilitation. He now has a gastrostomy tube. He has not found acceptable strategies for managing: 1) social occasions where he cannot eat, and 2) the saliva he can no longer swallow. His solution has been to isolate himself. He is angry and depressed; his wife feels helpless.
>
> Dx: Social life associated with eating disrupted R/T ineffective strategies for managing poststroke dysphagia L/T withdrawal, social isolation, anger, and depression.
>
> Prog: The dysphagia is permanent. The patient is an intelligent confident person, with a strong ego and a sense of humor. His wife is supportive of him. He has a strong network of friends. **IF** he can accept treatment that helps him to discover and utilize strategies and scripts for managing social situations with aplomb and some degree of humor, **THEN**

the prognosis is good for him to be able to rejoin his friends in their usual social activities in their homes if not in public places initially. His wife will support him in his efforts but will need to follow his lead rather than take the initiative herself.

Types of Outcomes

Several types of outcomes are possible with diagnosed nursing problems. Within these types of outcomes, one may predict either success, failure or, probably more commonly, some level of success between the two extremes.

Prevention

One possible outcome is avoidance of a problem entirely due to early identification of risk factors and introduction of timely risk reduction measures or preventive nursing actions. Conversely, the goal may be to prevent occurrence of a problem but the prognosis may be poor for achieving the desired outcome. For example:

Dx: Potential for impaired parenting R/T being a 16-year-old with deficits in knowledge and experience in infant care and lack of family support.

Prog: Prognosis for preventing impaired parenting is poor for this young girl based on her unwillingness to use resources for gaining knowledge and skills and lack of a usable support system. The school has a program on parenting, but the girl does not wish to use it, feels no need for the information, and is dropping out of school next week. She lacks insight into the challenges of parenting and feels that loving the infant will take care of everything. She has some difficulty with reading and has a limited vocabulary. She feels that her older "bright and pretty" sister is more loved by her parents and that she is particularly unwanted now because of the pregnancy and difficulties it is causing for the family. Her parents and sister are unaccepting of her pregnancy and her decision to go through with it and keep the child. The boy, identified by the girl as the biological father, claims he may not be the father and refuses any contact with her since she informed him of the pregnancy.

Delay or Minimization of Problem or Dysfunction

Another possible outcome is the occurrence of an expected problem but at a later time or in smaller magnitude than might normally be expected. Often this is the result of early recognition of the risks followed by treatment or other deterrents. For example:

Dx: Risk of contractures of joints on left side R/T new left hemiplegia with left hemianopsia & neglect of left half of body 2° CVA.

Prog: Immediate prognosis good for minimizing contractures because of skilled specialized nursing staff and the prompt, regular range of motion schedules, teaching the patient to turn his head to the left side and deliberately recognize his affected side.

Long term prognosis less promising. Wife seems ready to learn the activities and seeks to help; however, she appears to be a nonassertive person. Family reports patient has been dominant in the family. Loss of insight & judgment associated with left CVA plus vision deficits and inability to transfer learning from one situation to another 2° effects of CVA may restrict ongoing rehabilitation after discharge.

Resolution of Diagnosed Problems

The term "cure" tends to be associated with pathology. So perhaps the term "resolution" is more appropriate in describing the outcome of bringing a diagnosed nursing problem to a satisfactory conclusion. For example:

Dx: Impaired individual coping with required modifications in patterns of daily living R/T lack of knowledge and experience needed to live effectively with newly diagnosed insulin dependent diabetes.

Prog: Prognosis good that within months this patient and family will incorporate diabetic lifestyle into patterns of living in an effective and satisfying way. Patient has access to diabetic clinic including nurse specialists & dieticians as well as physicians. Classes and clearly written materials are available. The shock-denial phase of adaptation was a short one, and the patient has both the capacity and desire to learn but may have expectations that working knowledge and expertise will come faster than is realistic. A diabetic support group is available for both patient and family members. Initial monitoring suggests that the patient is not a brittle diabetic. Vision and muscular coordination have no current limitations—handles insulin injections efficiently. Funds and insurance are adequate for supplies, equipment, and food. Modification of usual meal patterns and family eating are being openly discussed. Anticipates that learning to handle the stresses and demands of work as they may affect her blood sugar may take time; is able to discuss them and engage in problem solving.

By way of contrast, another person with the same change in health status and requirements for change in lifestyle could have a poor prognosis for integration of these new demands into daily living. The denial response might be prolonged and continue to block attention to needed knowledge and skills as well as devalue their importance. The health care system might not have as many support elements; intellectual capacity for learning may be less; finances and insurance could be inadequate; family and home environment could be extremely nonsupportive; demands of the work situation might regularly cause fluctuations in blood sugar.

Improvement or Remission

Diagnosed phenomena in the nursing domain may show temporary improvement for a time or seem to disappear even though the underlying situation is still present.

Dx: Difficulty in obtaining entry-level employment and own health insurance R/T history of childhood leukemia and no longer being covered by parents' insurance.

Prog: Problem currently in remission. Through counseling on strategies for being a cancer survivor, patient obtained a job and was able to gain insurance during an "open" period. The difficulty will recur each time the patient seeks a different job more suited to his career goals and capabilities (Carnevali and Reiner, 1990).

Chronic diseases with fluctuating courses, such as bipolar mood disorders or multiple sclerosis generate patterns of remission and exacerbation that require major adjustments in managing daily living. Nursing recognition of a prognosis involving fluctuating phenomena is important. Appropriate treatment to assist patients and their families to manage fluctuating problems in remission and recurrence can be an important support to their well-being.

Stabilization

Some diagnosed nursing problems do not lend themselves to either prevention or resolution—they continue. Their ongoing pattern may be that of fluctuation or a downward trend. However, prognostic variables and data in the situation suggest that it may be possible to help those involved to achieve a reasonably steady state that will be more comfortable. The problem will continue, but fluctuations and deterioration may be minimized, at least for a time. For example:

Dx: Ineffective family coping with fluctuations in role requirements and relationships of family members R/T mother's periodic periods of dysfunction 2° multiple sclerosis.

Prog: Prognosis for stabilization is good. The adults have a good understanding of the pathology and the family dynamics involved. The daughters (10 and 12) are old enough and capable of understanding many of the issues. There is an established pattern of openness in communication. The family is willing to engage in periodic family councils to review the situation and the strategies that are effective and those that are ineffective or not satisfying for each. A nurse in the clinic is available for ongoing support and to teach the communication skills of giving feedback in ways that will be useful, not harmful. They seem to be open to learning strategies for dealing with the uncertainty of the situation.

Deterioration-Palliation

Some diagnosed nursing problems are destined to get worse in spite of any nursing treatment that can be employed. When this prognosis is made, treatment is directed toward support and palliation. The nurse seeks to help such patients and those who share their daily living to manage as effectively, as comfortably, and as satisfyingly as circumstances permit. For example:

Dx: Deteriorating lifestyle R/T homelessness, poverty, chronic schizophrenia and lack of support systems.

Prog: Prognosis poor for holding on to recent gains from improved nutrition and compliance with medication regimen through support of community health nurse. He has residual emotional "scars" and mistrust of people in bureaucracies from his early life in a series of abusive foster homes and placement in mental institutions. He "feels lonely" without his voices that used to keep him company before the medication caused them to disappear. Current pressures of life without home, money, or stable support system are forces that would seem to make relapse likely (case from Smith and Lunsford, 1990).

Palliation could include helping him to make use of some community resources, such as drop in centers (for support, laundry, and showers) and missions for meals. It could also include informing individuals in the community resources about the possibility that the patient may deteriorate and discussing strategies for continuing to work with him.

The ultimate outcome of a diagnosed problem can range from complete success in prevention, resolution, or stabilization to the opposite—failure to prevent, delay, or minimize, failure to resolve or stabilize, and failure to palliate or bring comfort and support as the condition worsens. These, of course, are the extremes in outcomes. Within an individual diagnosis and prognosis, outcomes usually fall somewhere in between. Having a realistic, data-supported prognostic outcome becomes crucial to planning for treatment. Each prognosis requires a different form of nursing treatment arising from a solid knowledge base associated with effective therapy for that outcome. The conceptual framework and knowledge base associated with integrating risk reduction behavior into daily living is different from that involved in palliation and support in an inevitably deteriorating situation.

It is important that the nurse's prognosis reflect reality, supported by data on appropriate prognostic variables. Nurses wish that outcomes would be positive as they care for patients and their families—that every case would have a happy ending. Unfortunately, life does not always work that way. Realistically, some situations will get worse, some preventable situations will not be prevented, some families will avoid or ignore available treatment, and some treatment will be ineffective or only partially effective. There will be positive prognoses, negative prognoses, and many that fall in between.

See *Exercise Set 1* for activities to identify nursing prognoses.

Trajectory

Prognosis deals with the course of events as well as outcomes. Characteristics of the course of events include what is expected to happen, the direction of change, and the pattern or rate of change. This can be called the trajectory.

Trajectories associated with different outcomes can vary. The onset of an expected problem may be delayed for a short or a long time. The trajectory for resolution or deterioration in a problem may be rapid or slow. Some changes may occur so slowly that they are not recognized by the patient or those closest to the situation unless baseline and ongoing evaluation data are used to concretely identify change. The pattern of change may appear as continuous change or be characterized by fluctuations and plateaus. Samples of trajectories for change are shown in Figure 4-2.

It is important for nurses to carefully consider the anticipated pattern and trajectory of change or lack of change as a basis for setting realistic goals and evaluation of response to treatment. This clinical judgment is also important for patients in order to help them adapt their expectations, daily living and allocation of resources to the anticipated course of events.

See *Exercise Set 2* for activities to recognize contingencies on prognoses.

Contingent Prognoses

Most prognoses are not cut and dried. Many are conditional in that they depend upon a variety of uncertain variables. When this is the case, the prognosis is stated in terms of the qualifiers **IF–THEN**. For example: **IF** this occurs **THEN** the prognosis should be good (see example, pp. 81–82). **IF** something fails to occur or new negative influences enter the picture, **THEN** the prognosis will be poor. Further, because of all of the variables that surround a nursing prognosis, they can be quite changeable. Therefore, it is wise to reassess the data if the patient's or family's response does not match the original prognosis.

See *Exercise Set 3* for activities to determine prognostic trajectory.

Realistic Data-supported Prognoses

It is much easier to deal with prognoses that leave the nurse and clients happy and satisfied. It is much harder to make and live with prognoses where outcomes leave patients and families feeling unhappy and dissatisfied and nurses feeling powerless, unsuccessful, frustrated, and depressed. Effective goal setting, treatment, evalua-

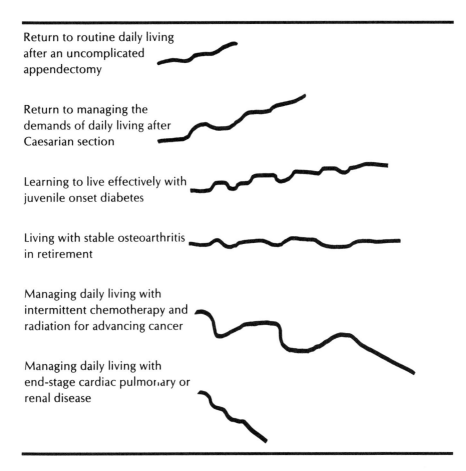

Return to routine daily living
after an uncomplicated
appendectomy

Return to managing the
demands of daily living after
Caesarian section

Learning to live effectively with
juvenile onset diabetes

Living with stable osteoarthritis
in retirement

Managing daily living with
intermittent chemotherapy and
radiation for advancing cancer

Managing daily living with
end-stage cardiac pulmonary or
renal disease

FIGURE 4-2   Examples of Trajectory in Nursing Prognosis

tion, and even caring depend upon professional honesty, not wishful thinking.
See *Exercise Set 7* for data based nursing prognoses.

The Perspective in Nursing Prognosis

Nursing prognosis deals with the likelihood that the patient or family will be able to
respond to the actual or potential health problem in such a way that:

■ Health, well-being, and effective functioning are promoted.
■ Daily living is as effectively managed as capacities, external resources, and daily
living permit.
■ The resultant quality of life is satisfying.

The Relationship of Nursing Prognosis to Medical Prognosis

It would seem reasonable to think that medical and nursing prognosis would move in the same direction—that when a medical prognosis is positive, the nursing prognosis would also be positive. Also, that the reverse would be true—a negative medical prognosis would automatically result in a negative nursing prognosis. This is not necessarily the case since medical and nursing prognoses address different problem areas. While the course of events and outcomes identified in the medical prognosis are factors in many nursing prognoses, they are not the only influences.

Negative Medical Prognoses and Positive Nursing Prognoses

Sometimes the medical prognosis for the pathology is that the condition will not get better or will worsen. Under these circumstances, many nurses still have seen situations in which the nursing prognosis for effective management of daily living and achieving satisfaction with the quality of life was a positive one. For example:

> A jazz saxophonist at the height of his career suffered a stroke and hemiplegia yet returned to performing professionally, using only one hand, and continued to win professional and audience respect for the caliber of his playing.

> An 8-year-old girl has cerebral palsy accompanied by seizures for which she receives medication. She has a vocabulary of a few words. She drowses frequently as a result of her medication. She lives with her mother and younger sister and next door to a caring grandmother. There are many adult family friends and children who visit the home and who readily accept her. She is a part of the family's activities inside and outside the home. She is always well groomed and attractive. The home and a van are adapted for her wheelchair. She attends a special education program in public school. She goes horseback riding each week in a program for handicapped children. Her medical prognosis is very limited, but her support system is superb and the quality of her life is as good as it possibly can be.

It is important to remember that pathophysiologic status is not synonymous with managing one's daily living as effectively as one's health status permits and finding satisfaction in it. Individuals who are dying in hospice settings, whose pain and other symptoms are managed, and whose support network remains close, often manage daily living with dying effectively and find some satisfactions.

Positive Medical Prognoses and Negative Nursing Prognoses

It would seem that a positive medical prognosis would assure that the patient and family would make a positive response to the illness experience and would manage their daily living effectively and with satisfaction. But this is not necessarily true. For example:

> A young man has been given a very positive prognosis that his treatment for testicular cancer has been highly successful. However, he remains hypervigilant about every sign and symptom, is unable to get health insurance, is unable to form satisfying relationships with women, feels alienated from people who have not had his illness experience, has no access to a support group. He is lonely and centers his daily living around the possibility of recurrence.

> A woman in her twenties had juvenile onset diabetes. She is disciplined in her diet, insulin injections, and self-monitoring. She builds her whole life around managing her diabetes. Her blood sugar is consistently well controlled and she shows no diabetic complications. However, she feels like she is living in a prison created by her diabetes and finds no satisfaction or joy in life.

It is possible to prevent, cure or control pathology and thus have a positive medical prognosis and at the same time have a negative nursing prognosis.

See *Exercise Set 4* comparing nursing with medical prognoses.

Risks in Prognosticating

A prognosis is a prediction, an educated guess, a possibility. It is not a certainty. It is based on patient data, on knowledge of previous clinical experiences or research associated with the phenomenon or problem, but it is still a clinical judgment with room for error. Often nurses in institutional work settings see only a small sample of the individual's and family's health situation. For example:

> A woman with bipolar mood disorder may have been managing daily living well. She has been stabilized on medications, and she and her family have made adjustments in their lifestyle. She has sustained both family responsibilities and a job. An uncontrolled cycling into mania results in a 3-week hospitalization where she is seen sleeping only a few hours per night, expressing grandiose beliefs, and behaving impulsively and seductively.

> If nurses fail to place this short episode into the context of previous effectiveness and adequacy of resources in living with her mood disorder, they may well generate an inaccurately negative prognosis.[1]

Like a diagnosis, a prognosis can take on a life of its own. It can become reality for the nurse, the patient, and the family. Goals, treatment, expectations, self-concept, and evaluation emerge from prognosis as well as diagnosis. Therefore, it is important that prognoses be as well-founded as possible.

---

[1]Case example offered by Jeffrey Thurston, RN, CS, MN.

Risks of an Inaccurate Positive Prognosis

What are the risks if a nurse makes an incorrect positive prognosis of response to the diagnosed situation? Goals and evaluation criteria are set for a positive outcome. Treatment is directed toward helping the patient or family to produce the expected outcome. When this outcome does not occur, frustration may occur, blame may be assigned to the patient or family, or a new diagnosis of noncompliance may be assigned. The nurse may feel ineffectual and guilty. The relationship with the patient and family may become less positive and therapeutic. For example:

> A woman in the advanced stage of AIDS was admitted with a 6-week history of anorexia, nausea, and progressive weight loss. The nurse's prognosis was that, with medical treatment and support in eating a nourishing diet, this pattern could be reversed. Based on this prognosis the goal was set that the patient would ingest 2500 calories per day including 60 gm of protein. The treatment included providing the patient with foods she said she enjoyed, at times she said her appetite was best, as attractively served as possible, with strong encouragement to eat. The woman did not or could not ingest the desired calories and protein. Nursing treatment of "encouragement to eat" became tinged with exasperation, frustration, threat, and guilt-producing behavior. The woman's nutritional status and eating behavior continued to deteriorate and nurses spent less time with her. As mutual frustration set in, their relationships became more superficial.

Prognostic expectations that are inappropriately high or positive place pressures on patients, families, and nurses to achieve these outcomes. When reality does not match the prediction, both patient and nurse can experience disappointment, frustration, anger, and guilt. If it seems that a prognosis may be erring on the positive side, it is important to reexamine the prognostic data in the situation. It may be appropriate to reassess the prognostic variables and make adjustments.

Risks of an Inappropriately Negative Prognosis

An inaccurate negative prognosis also can create problems, particularly for the patient and family. It can become a self-fulfilling prophecy. When a patient or family sense by the nurse's attitude or treatment that a negative outcome is anticipated, they can give up or fall in with the expectations and associated treatment. Nursing treatment can actually support a negative outcome. For example:

> In the case of the young girl with severe cerebral palsy and seizures, the nurses could have made a prognosis that her pathology and the side effects of the anticonvulsant medications made her incapable of benefiting from interaction with other children or from special education programs. A care plan for basic maintenance and sensory stimulation could have been developed with the mother, and the child could essentially have been relegated to the back bedroom rather than included in all family activities.

It is as important to be accurate about prognosis as it is to be accurate about diagnosis. Each one has a major influence on treatment, whether the judgments are made consciously or without awareness.

See *Exercise Set 5* for exercises in effects of inaccurate prognoses.

Elements in Making Prognostic Judgments

Just as there is a pattern of elements in diagnostic reasoning, there is also one in making prognostic judgments. This, too, involves information processing—combining data with knowledge and experience to arrive at clinical judgments, as shown in Display 4-1.

Identification of the Specific Diagnosis as Area for Prognosis

In order to develop an accurate prognosis, it is essential to begin with a specific diagnosis rather than a general diagnostic category. Using the NANDA category of

---

DISPLAY 4-1
ELEMENTS IN MAKING PROGNOSTIC JUDGMENTS

Identify the specific diagnosis for which a prognosis is to be determined.

Retrieve from long term memory:

Prognostic possibilities associated with this specific diagnosis (areas for change, outcomes, trajectory).
Variables that will influence these prognostic possibilities.
Observable or reportable data that would give evidence of the nature of the variables in the present situation.

Use the prognostic variables and associated findings as guides[a] for viewing the situation and assembling a prognostic database.

Analyze the prognostic data collected.

Make prognostic judgments.

If appropriate, discuss the prognosis for course of events and outcomes as well as the factors influencing prognosis with the person involved.

---

[a] An example of a prognostic observational guide that could be used to determine a prognosis for managing daily living with iatrogenic diarrhea is shown on pp. 93, 95–96 together with the data collected in a particular patient situation.

"Sleep Pattern Disturbance" (Carroll-Johnson, 1991, p. 380), one would move to more specific diagnoses:

Wakening at inappropriate hours R/T 8 hour change in time zone would have a prognosis of resolving itself within a week if the person has no other sleep disorder. This prognostic judgment is based on the underlying knowledge that it takes one day of readjustment for every hour of time change.

Prognosis for a parent's chronic sleep deprivation (Assousa and Wilson, 1991) R/T caregiving responsibilities for a child on a respirator will depend upon the child's response to the respirator and physiologic stability, the anxiety level of the caregiver, and the availability of someone trusted to take over the caregiving responsibilities at regular needed intervals.

Each of these diagnoses fall into the general category of sleep pattern disturbance, yet each has different prognostic variables.

Retrieval of Prognostic Possibilities and Factors Influencing Prognosis from Long Term Memory

In each diagnostic concept there is a portion dealing with recognition features that make diagnosis possible, but there is another portion containing knowledge needed to make prognostic judgments. The prognostic portion of the concept will contain knowledge about underlying dynamics of the phenomenon, and from that, the prognostic possibilities and the variables that will affect them. Knowledge and patient instances are retrieved from long term memory in the process of making prognostic judgments. An illustration of a sequence of this knowledge is shown in Figure 4-3. For example:

Nursing diagnostic area: Individual coping with requirements of daily living with iatrogenic diarrhea.

Underlying variables and mechanisms: Changes in tissue structure or physiology associated with this diarrhea; severity and predicted duration of the diarrhea; status of sphincter control to contain liquid stool; status of mobility and physical strength for getting to toilet facilities, removal of clothing, and care of perianal area; physical access to toilet facilities that accommodate to the time between the urge to defecate and the time when control is no longer possible; access to

Specific nursing diagnosis		Underlying variables and mechanisms		Prognostic variables

FIGURE 4-3   Knowledge Needed in Order to Make Prognostic Nursing Judgments

protective clothing; ability to understand the relationship between diet and diarrhea and willingness to modify eating patterns to reduce roughage and increase fluids and potassium in diet; patterns in daily living that affect ways of managing discomfort and toileting; self-concept associated with bowel control.

Prognostic variables: Poor prognosis is associated with:

- Severe, prolonged diarrhea.
- Decreased sphincter control.
- Restricted mobility and strength.
- Difficult access to toilet facilities (distance, stairs, number of other people who must also use the toilet).
- Patterns in daily living that require travel, work, or social activities where leaving to go to the toilet is difficult and bowel incontinence is intolerable.
- Restricted joint flexibility or muscular strength to permit rapid removal of clothing prior to defecation.
- Lack of physical or mental capacity to properly cleanse and protect the perianal area to minimize skin breakdown.
- Lack of ability to understand the relationship between diet and diarrhea; lack of willingness or ability to change to a low residue diet, and increase fluids and potassium in diet.
- Lack of access to protective garments or unwillingness to use them.
- Difficulties in finding appropriate transportation when leaving the home.
- Equating bowel incontinence with a negative self-image and feelings of shame rather than acknowledging an unavoidable, treatment-caused physiological state.
- Lack of adequate laundry facilities or services or adequate amount of clothing to wear when soiled clothing is being laundered.
- Lack of knowledge about how to safely launder clothing soiled with feces.
- Inadequate hand washing patterns.
- Lack of understanding and support from those who share daily living, e.g., dietary changes, reason for the diarrhea, modifying their own behavior to allow access to the toilet as needed, changes in the sexual interests or capacity of the patient.

It can be seen that the capacity to make accurate prognostic judgments in the nursing domain can only be as good as the base of knowledge and clinical experience that can be retrieved from long term memory to serve as an observational guide in viewing the presenting patient situation.

Collection of Data Using the Prognostic Observational Guide

When one has an understanding of the underlying dynamics in the diagnosed patient situation and can identify variables affecting the course of events and outcomes, it is possible to gather data to make a prognosis.

The Place of Medical Data in the Nursing Prognosis

The nursing prognostic database often includes medical data and associated knowledge. This would include the medical diagnosis, factors influencing its occurrence, structural changes, pathophysiological changes, and effects or predicted effects of treatment.

Medical knowledge and data are needed when the nursing prognosis involves prevention. For example:

> If the nursing diagnosis addresses a person's human response to the potential problem of acquiring a communicable disease (prevention), one of the areas of knowledge needed is the nature of the organism, routes of transmission, and any currently available means of prevention or minimizing risk.
>
>> If the problem is a risk of acquiring AIDS, the focus would be on daily living and lifestyle involving placement of physical barriers and on behavioral actions to prevent contact between the body fluids of infected and noninfected individuals. The time between infection and clinical manifestations may be long. The infected person can be identified by a positive HIV serum test months after the infection occurs. (Altman, 1991).

> If the nursing diagnosis involves risk of ineffectiveness or burnout in a spouse or parent serving as caregiver (Gaynor, 1990), then medical data are needed about the health status of both caregiver and patient. Concerning the patient, knowledge is needed about nature, intensity, and duration of care needed. For the care provider, one may need data on any health problem that will interfere with the functional capacities to provide the needed care. For example:
>
>> The patient may be a heavy man who has had a stroke and requires physical assistance with change of position and ambulation. How much chronic deficit in mobility is predicted? Does his wife, who is his caregiver, have any health problems that prevent or impair her ability to provide this assistance at present and for the duration of the predicted mobility deficit?

Medical knowledge is also needed when the nursing prognosis involves a situation where pathology is present. Again, there is a need to know the nature of any changes in structure or physiological functioning, the desired and iatrogenic effects of the medical therapy, and the medical prognosis. For example:

> A previously healthy, nonsmoking 28-year-old man is diagnosed as having pneumococcal pneumonia. Structural changes in the lungs are those of an inflammatory response. The pathophysiology involves impaired gaseous exchange with resultant hypoxemia and hyperventilation plus a generalized body response of high fever, fatigue, cough, and pleuritic pain. The medical treatment given is Penicillin G procaine. Initial clinical response to treatment is expected within 24–48 hours. Complete clearance of the infiltrate in the lungs is expected to take weeks.

That same pneumonia in someone who is elderly or who has a compromised immune system would be much less likely to quickly and completely respond to medical treatment. The presence of an oxygen deficit, fatigue, and pleuritic pain will present different challenges to the functional capacities and external resources in these two cases and will affect the assessment of nursing prognostic variables. An older person or one with a compromised immune system will require adjustments in activities, demands, and environment for daily living over a longer period of time and need more external resources for a longer duration. This brings up different prognostic variables than those in the initial example where the medical situation is acute but of a relatively short duration.

Assessing Nursing Prognostic Variables

When knowledge about the relevant prognostic variables has been retrieved from long term memory, it is possible to use this knowledge to direct data collection. One sorts out the prognostic data that are available from a variety of sources. The following example illustrates the previously described observational guide of prognostic variables associated with managing daily living effectively with iatrogenic diarrhea.

Mr. Jones is a 45-year-old who has been having pelvic radiation treatment and is experiencing iatrogenic diarrhea. He needs to continue to work in his present job in order to support his family and maintain his health insurance. He has been employed as a short haul truck driver with the same company for 10 years and has been on sick leave for treatment of his malignancy.

Status of diarrhea:	3–5 liquid stools daily. Some cramping. Occasional urgency. Diarrhea may continue as a long term side effect of radiation.
Sphincter control:	Variable.
Toilet accessibility:	Limited to truck stops and gas stations, often with many miles between.
Travel:	Regular trips of 100–400 miles, 5–6 days per week.
Joint flexibility:	No problem.
Muscular strength:	Some fatigue, but sufficient strength to manage clothing removal for defecation.
Ability for perianal hygiene:	Understands and is consistent. Carries packets of baby wipes plus ointment in truck for cleansing and protection.
Diet:	Understands and tries to eat low-residue diet. Some difficulty in roadside restaurants. Knows

	high potassium, low residue foods and eats them.
Fluid replacement:	Carries bottles of fluids in truck.
Protective garments:	Reluctant to use them. Wears chino pants and pads for leakage. Carries extra pants, pads, and underwear.
Emotional response to bowel incontinence:	Uses humor to deal with episodes of fecal incontinence. "What can't be helped must be lived with. Right now I can't always control it—but I manage."
Laundry:	Carries soiled clothing in plastic bag. Wife does the family laundry and gives evidence of understanding safe laundry practices with fecal material.
Hand washing:	Has been shown and return-demonstrated effective hand washing technique. Knows importance in not causing himself and others additional health problems.
Support system:	His wife reports that his own attitude and acceptance make it easy for others to remain close to him. The family has been close and supportive during treatment and continues this way. Conversations with patient indicate a strong support network.

Analysis of Prognostic Data and Determination of Prognosis

When data have been sorted out, it is possible to make a current judgment as to the course of events and outcomes in the diagnostic area. Since nursing diagnoses are more transitory than medical diagnoses, it follows that nursing prognoses may also be more subject to change than medical prognoses.

Using the data assembled in the case of the truck driver, the nurse would make the judgment that, for now:

The patient is managing the challenges of living with diarrhea very well. Often the diarrhea associated with radiation abates within weeks of completion of the treatment. However, it is also possible for it to continue as a long term iatrogenic aftereffect.

It would be wise to gather fresh data at a later date should the challenges of managing daily living with diarrhea continue at this level of severity.

Discussion of the Prognosis With the Person

It is both ethical and a part of therapy that clinical judgments made about prognosis be discussed with the person if it is appropriate. Some individuals cannot participate in prognostic judgments, e.g., persons with decreased levels of consciousness, with cognitive deficits, or extreme physiological instability. Some patients may lack the capacity for insight to consider prognosis, e.g., those who have impaired judgment due to a CVA on the left side, patients in acute drug intoxication or psychoses, or those who are in the denial stage of adaptation to a new diagnosis. Others may be more comfortable with uncertainty (Mishel, 1988; 1990).

For most individuals (patients or others) for whom prognoses are made, a discussion of the prognostic variables, course of events and possible outcomes are a right and a necessary foundation for participation in managing the situation. For example:

> "Tommy, you're about to have a new experience for a 6-year-old tomorrow when you have your surgery. You told me that your mom has read to you about what it's like to come to the hospital and have an operation. You and your brother even had a make-believe hospital and surgery. You certainly ask good questions about everything. You said you knew it wouldn't be a piece of cake, that your tummy would be hurting afterwards, but that we'd all work to keep you as comfortable as we can. Your mom will be here and so will I. Do you feel pretty ready to manage it?"

Where there is a negative prognosis—where the challenges to coping involve either increasing demands or diminishing functional capacities or external resources—it is possible to talk with the person in terms of the challenges they face and options for managing. For example:

Diagnosis: Incipient burnout R/T care demands of wife with Alzheimer's & his functional limitations 2° coronary artery disease.

Prognosis: Poor, based on his total preoccupation with his wife's care, growing distress over her behavior, his inability to link her behavior to the pathology, his progressing coronary artery disease, chronic sleep deprivation, lack of respite, lack of participation in Alzheimer's support group, loss of former social activities, geographic distance from other family members and limited finances.

Sample RN discussion of prognosis with person: "Mr. Burns, I'm concerned about how you are going to continue to manage as Mrs. Burns' Alzheimer's disease continues. You have been such a close couple and you've been totally devoted to her and her care for months now. Given your own heart problem, it can't be easy maintaining the 24-hour surveillance she is requiring. . . . Unless it is possible to get some reliable, regular respite and some support, I am worried that you could become ill, too. Is there any way you can get others to take over some of the time so that you can get some rest and some time away from the demands?"

Prognostic discussions should be undertaken in a **timely manner.** Timeliness can be determined by the demands of the situation or by the readiness of the patient to deal with the prognosis.

Sometimes, prognostic judgment concerns human response to an upcoming situation such as an upcoming medical treatment (as illustrated by the example of Tommy above) or needing to make important personal or business decisions when the patient is the only one or the one best able to make them and has only a limited time within which to make the decision. Then the timing of the prognostic discussion is determined by the situation rather than the readiness of the patient. For example:

> For a single mother in her thirties, death from ovarian cancer is only days away. She has two children, ages 4 and 6. She still speaks of getting better and expects to recover. Several relatives have indicated a willingness to assume responsibility for the children; yet it seems that the mother who knows them and her children best should be the one to make the choice as to their placement and to formalize this decision so as to minimize stress for the children. The nurse could talk about this prognosis-based decision as a type of insurance policy. One doesn't always use an insurance policy, but it adds to one's security to have it available.

Often the nurse makes a decision to engage in the prognostic discussion when the patient is ready. Such discussions can involve both a positive or negative prognosis. Some patients for whom illness produces secondary gains may not be ready to hear a positive prognosis for improvement in their ability to manage the demands of life. Many patients are unready to learn about increasing challenges and difficulties to be faced. For the nurse, sharing prognostic judgments can be a foundation for nursing treatment. It needs to be done in a way that helps rather than diminishes the person's capacity to participate in the health-related situation.

See *Exercise Set 6* for activities using the elements in prognostic thinking.

The Place of Prognostic Judgments in the Plan of Care

At present, nurses' plans of care tend to feature diagnoses, goals, treatment, and evaluation. Prognostic judgments are not documented. Still, written or unwritten, prognostic judgments should have an obvious influence on goals, treatment, and evaluation.

Influence of Nursing Prognoses on Goals

Goals tend to represent desired outcomes—the ideal. Certainly, goals or outcome criteria associated with standard care plans take this approach (Reiner, 1988; Carpenito, 1989, 1990). Prognoses, when they are valid and accurate, represent reality as far as human judgment permits. Sometimes desired outcomes and prognosis are congruent. This happy agreement tends to occur when the prognosis is a positive one, and fortunately, this is often the case.

On the other hand, there are times when an ideal outcome is not realistic. Then the desired outcomes need to be tempered with the reality of a valid prognosis. **A useful, realistic goal needs to reflect a valid prognosis.** Where a prognosis is less than ideal, a nurse and the person who is involved need to work to achieve some kind of consensus as to goals that are realistically achievable and desirable, given a guarded prognostic judgment regarding available functional capacities, requirements of daily living, and external resources that can be mobilized. Nurses need to acquire skill in making useful, acceptable goals when there is a negative prognosis. It is a much more difficult task than goal setting where outcome and trajectory are positive.

A prognosis may not be documented as such on a clinical record, however, it should certainly be apparent in a realistic goal statement.

Prognosis as an Influence on Nursing Treatment

Nursing treatment is not the same when it is addressing such differing goals as seeking to prevent, minimize or delay, cure or resolve, manage life with remissions, stabilize, or manage life in deteriorating situations. Thus, all elements of prognosis need to be considerations in planning treatment—the areas, outcomes, and trajectory. Each can and should affect nursing treatment.

Prognosis as a Consideration in Evaluation

Evaluation has close ties to desired or expected outcomes and the nursing actions undertaken to enable the person to achieve those outcomes. The trajectory of change is also important in considering timing for gathering evaluative data.

Prognostic Outcomes and Evaluation

Outcomes that have been predicted for a patient determine the criteria for evaluation. If prognosis suggests that a phenomenon or event can be *prevented,* the outcome criteria will be that it does not appear. If a dysfunction or difficulty cannot be prevented but only *delayed or minimized,* then the criteria must address the appearance of the phenomenon or event at a time later than would be anticipated or of lesser magnitude than would have been the case without nursing intervention. For example:

> Stiffness is a normal human response to pathology associated with Parkinson's disease. Yet a daily regimen of stretching and range of motion can sometimes delay or decrease the stiffness (Linde, 1993).

If a problem can be *resolved/cured*, then obviously manifestations of the difficulty or inadequate or impaired functioning will disappear in the time interval that is predicted. For example:

Newly diagnosed diabetics whose prognosis suggests that they will be able to resolve the difficulties of adapting to living with diabetes cannot be expected to gain all the needed working knowledge, skills, insights, and adaptive strategies in weeks. The prognostic pattern here usually is a matter of months.

Similarly, outcomes associated with human responses to managing life with *remission and recurrence* will need to be adapted to the anticipated time pattern and the challenges to human response associated with the significance of the recurrence. For example:

Recurrence of a treatable urinary tract infection or a predicted moderate allergic response will create less challenge to human responses and daily living than will recurrence of a life-threatening condition such as a metastatic malignancy or a pneumonia in an immunosuppressed individual.

When the nurse is evaluating response to goal and treatment to *stabilize* human responses and daily living, then outcome criteria would be lack of change rather than change. And finally, when the treatment is to help an individual to manage a *deteriorating* situation, the evaluative criteria will address satisfaction with quality of life and managing the requirements of daily living with diminishing resources.

Prognostic Trajectory and Collection of Evaluative Data

Prognosis affects not only the focus of evaluation but also the points in time when one collects data for evaluation of response to treatment. Some phenomena will respond rapidly, and evaluative data can be collected shortly after treatment has been initiated. For example:

The prognosis for preoperative teaching to affect postoperative behavior will be measured as soon as the patient is conscious after surgery and is asked to engage in the behaviors taught, e.g., deep breathing, coughing, and turning.

The trajectory for another situation may be one of slow progress—small gains followed by plateaus of no change, or low points and then small gains again. Strauss (1989) for example describes plateaus and periods of change in the trajectory of schizophrenia. In such situations responses will be timed to note the duration of "no change plateaus" and the amount of change when it occurs.

The timing of data collection for evaluative purposes is extremely important. If one collects data on response before that response has had time to occur, the findings will be that it did not occur. But that would be wrong—they had not occurred *yet*.

Prognosis and Evaluation of Extent of Change

Prognosis assists in determining the extent of change that should be anticipated. In some problems that lend themselves to quick resolution, one should be prepared to look for large amounts of change associated with rapid disappearance of the difficulty. In other situations the amounts of change, either of improvement or deterioration, will be very small. For example:

> Some patients who have had strokes rapidly regain mobility and functional capacities on the affected side but may have other deficits that respond much more slowly—over months. The changes in these more chronic functional deficits and related problems in managing daily living will occur in much smaller increments than the initial response.

Setting criteria that dictate greater change than the prognosis suggests would be a poor evaluative strategy.

It can be seen that prognosis is a critical feature in undertaking evaluation. It can be used to determine realistic outcome criteria, timing of data collection for evaluative purposes and determination of the amount of change that can be expected.

See *Exercise Set 7* for activities associated with integrating prognosis into plans of care.

Summary

It is not enough in planning nursing care to use the medical prognosis as the structure for goals and treatment. Nursing's different perspective requires that nursing prognostic judgments be the basis for nursing goals, treatment, and evaluation. Predicting the future is an uncertain process and carries some risk for error that could result in grave consequences for the person being evaluated. It is important, therefore, to have an adequate knowledge base (both theoretical and experiential) and to gather a sound database as a foundation for prognostic judgments. Appropriate exploration of the prognostic judgment and the database with the person can be a source of validation as well as an element in the treatment plan.

Prognoses can be as useful a therapeutic tool in nursing as they are in medicine, despite the reality that our current body of knowledge rarely separates out this feature. For multiple examples of attempts to structure knowledge in this way, see Carnevali and Reiner, 1990. In the meantime, it is possible to utilize present knowledge and experience to develop an adequate, usable basis for making prognostic judgments that will form a reasonable structure for nursing goals, treatment, and evaluation for those we treat.

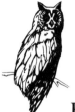

Exercises on Prognostic Judgments

Set 1 □ Prognostic Outcomes[2]

1. A. Recall situations where the person was well and your prognostic outcome was that potential threats to health could be prevented from occurring because of nursing interventions.
   B. Find situations where the patient is ill or dysfunctional and your prognosis is that a further health problem or complication can be prevented because of nursing treatment.
   C. Find patient situations where the potential problem seems not to be preventable but could be delayed or minimized by nursing treatment.
2. Find situations where you predict that a diagnosed nursing problem can be resolved by nursing treatment.
3. Find situations where you predict recurring periods of improvement and difficulties in managing health problems or daily living with health problems.
4. Find situations where you predict fluctuations in ability to manage the health problem and associated daily living that could be stabilized with nursing treatment.
5. Find situations in which you predict unavoidable deterioration in functioning, management of daily living, or external resources, a prognosis where nursing treatment would be supportive and palliative rather than restorative.

Set 2 □ Contingent Prognoses

1. Find situations in which you see the prognostic outcome as being clear-cut or with little chance that intervening circumstances or treatment can change it. Think of both positive and negative ones.
2. Find IF–THEN prognostic situations where IF certain events, responses, external factors, or nursing treatment take place, THEN one prognostic outcome is predicted to occur, while IF other events, conditions, treatment, responses occur, THEN a different outcome will be predicted.
3. Write down contingent prognoses on one or more of your patients, caregivers, family members, etc. Observe the factors that actually occurred that influenced the course of events and the actual outcome. Compare it to your prediction.

---

[2]Note: While the exercise instructions may specify patient situation (for sake of brevity) these exercises can also focus on caregivers, family members, groups, or community.

Set 3 □ Prognostic Trajectory

1. Identify patients you care for in whom the course of events, both in direction and rate of change, varies. Think about the factors in the situation that influence both direction and rate of change. Look at both short and long term trajectories. Plot the trajectories.

Set 4 □ Comparison of Medical and Nursing Prognoses

1. Identify patient situations in which the medical prognoses are negative, yet the person is managing the difficulties effectively, making the nursing prognosis a positive one. Identify other situations where both medical and nursing prognoses are negative—pathology is worsening, and management of the health experience and daily living with it also is very poor.
2. Identify situations in which the person is complying with the medical treatment or health care regimen. The medical prognosis for prevention, cure, or stabilization is excellent but the resultant quality of life in one or more areas is negative or unsatisfying to the person, and therefore, the nursing prognosis is negative. Identify other situations where both the medical and nursing prognoses are good.
3. Find situations in which a nursing diagnosis and prognosis can be made when no medical diagnosis or prognosis is involved. Identify patients, caregivers, or family members for whom you make a nursing diagnosis and prognosis not linked to medical diagnosis or care.
4. Select one or more of your current patients. Identify the medical prognosis and make a nursing prognosis. Follow up to determine the accuracy of each prognosis.

Set 5 □ Effects of Inaccurate Prognostication

1. Identify a patient situation in which nursing prognosis or outcome (thought or formalized into writing) is thought to be good, and with treatment being directed toward that outcome but the patient or situation is not meeting nursing expectations. Is the nursing behavior or attitude changing toward the patient, family or others? If so, in what way? Are these changes therapeutic for the patient and family or not? In what way?
2. Recall a situation in which the nursing prognosis (expectations) were that the person would not respond to the health situation in ways to produce a positive outcome, with treatment and attitudes overtly or subtly supporting this expectation. However, the individual surprised everyone and managed at a much higher level than expected. Did nursing care or attitudes create any barriers or unnecessary difficulties?

Set 6 □ Use of the Elements of Prognostic Thinking

1. A. Select a nursing diagnostic area you are using with one of your current patients. Make a list of all of the variables in the patient's situation that could

affect the outcome. Indicate whether they are positive or negative influences on the prognosis. Consider the nature and requirements of past, present, and future daily living (activities, events, self-expectations, demands of others, environmental demands, values, and beliefs), functional capacities and external resources. If a family member or caregiver is also closely involved, identify a diagnostic area for this person as well and make a comparable list.

B. Use the lists as data collection guides and gather data on prognostic variables about the patient and the family member or caregiver. Notice how the nursing prognosis for each individual or group affects that of the others.

C. Collect information on any physiological or pathophysiological status that is relevant and any physician diagnostic or treatment activities that will be positive or negative factors for these two prognostic areas. Remember that medical activities and their effects can be a factor in family or caregiver prognoses as well as that of the patient.

D. Make a nursing prognosis for a patient, family member, or caregiver. Then develop a script about how you might discuss this with the patient and the family member or caregiver. Remember that this discussion should be therapeutic and not destructive to them. Role-play it with a colleague and get feedback on how the interaction was experienced. Revise your script and replay it. Reevaluate. Did you need to modify your prognosis based on additional feedback in the role-playing.

E. As soon as you feel comfortable and skilled from having practiced this interaction with nonpatients, try the experience of discussing a nursing prognosis with a patient or family member/caregiver.

Set 7 ☐ Integrating Prognoses Into Plans of Care

1. Select two patients—one for whom the nursing diagnosis is quite general and another where it is quite specific. How does the specificity of the nursing diagnosis help in developing accurate nursing prognoses? Why do you need a specific nursing diagnosis before you can engage in prognostic thinking? Look at the documented nursing assessment. Can you get all of the prognostic data you need from the data used to develop the diagnosis? If not, what particular categories seem to be missing? Where will you go to obtain the additional data? If you need examples of a wide variety of prognostic variables and types of data, see *The Cancer Experience: Nursing Diagnosis and Management* (Carnevali and Reiner, 1990).

2. A. Select a patient for whom there are a database and diagnosis. Identify the goals that you would set for this patient and family. Then examine the prognoses for the diagnosis. What, if any, are the differences between your prognoses and the goals or desired outcomes you set? How can you integrate your prognoses and goals?

   B. What kind of goals can you set when the nursing prognosis is quite negative (unremitting deterioration of the situation)? Consider your satisfaction and that of the patient when achievable goals are set within a deteriorating situation.

3. A. Identify ways in which nursing prognoses influence nursing treatment decisions.

   B. How might prognostic trajectories and outcomes in a specific case differ from the stated "desired outcomes" of a standard care plan for that condition or situation?

   C. Select a patient whose diagnosis permits use of a standard plan of care that includes desired outcomes. Make a specific nursing diagnosis within the general diagnostic area specified in the plan. Be certain to individualize it with this patient's data. From this diagnosis determine the prognostic variables, gather data on the prognostic variables in this specific situation, make a prognostic judgment, and identify the predicted trajectory and outcome. Plan your nursing treatment to take these into account. Compare your individualized treatment based on the specific diagnosis and prognosis with the treatment of the standard plan. How are they the same? How did they differ? If they are different, what difference do you think it would make to the patient or family if adjustments in the standard care plan were not made?

4. A. Identify the ways in which prognostic judgments about trajectory and outcomes influence evaluation of response to nursing treatment, e.g., areas to be evaluated, expected rate of change, expected changes, timing of evaluation, data to be used, and outcome standards.

   B. Select two patients facing relatively comparable health situations but who have the potential to manage them in different ways. Make a prognosis involving trajectory and outcome for each. Plan the evaluation based on your activities in Exercise 4A, e.g., when data are collected, what data are collected and rate and type of change (or lack of change) expected in this situation compared to the standard.

References

ALTMAN G: Infectious disorders of the blood and acquired immunodeficiency syndrome (AIDS). In Patrick M, Woods S, Craven R, Rokosky J, Bruno P (eds): *Medical-Surgical Nursing: Pathophysiological Concepts*. 2nd ed. Philadelphia: J.B. Lippincott, 1991, pp. 938–949.

ASSOUSA S, WILSON N: Validation of sleep pattern disturbance. Abstract in Carroll-Johnson R (ed): *Classification of Nursing Diagnoses: Proceedings of the Ninth Conference North American Nursing Diagnosis Association*. Philadelphia: J.B. Lippincott, 1991.

CARNEVALI D, REINER A: *The Cancer Experience: Nursing Diagnosis and Management*. Philadelphia: J.B. Lippincott, 1990.

CARPENITO L:. *Nursing Care Plans and Documentation: Nursing Diagnoses and Collaborative Problems*. Philadelphia: J.B. Lippincott, 1990.

CARPENITO L: *Nursing Diagnosis: Application to Clinical Practice*. 4th ed. Philadelphia: J.B. Lippincott, 1991.

CARROLL-JOHNSON R: *Classification of Nursing Diagnoses: Proceedings of the Ninth Conference, North American Nursing Diagnosis Association*. Philadelphia: J.B. Lippincott, 1991.

GAYNOR S: The long haul: The effects of home care on caregivers. *Image: Journal of Nursing Scholarship* 22(4):208–212, 1990.

LINDE M: Parkinsonism. In Carnevali D, Patrick M (eds): *Nursing Management for the Elderly*. 3rd ed. Philadelphia: J.B. Lippincott, 1993.

MISHEL M: Reconceptualization of the uncertainty in illness theory. *Image: Journal of Nursing Scholarship* 22(4):256–262, 1990.

MISHEL M: Uncertainty in illness. *Image: Journal of Nursing Scholarship* 20:255, 1988.

REINER A: *Manual of Patient Care Standards*. Rockville, MD: Aspen Publishers, 1988. Annual supplements 89, 90, 91, 92.

SMITH L, LUNSFORD B: Mental health needs of homeless persons. In MacFarland G, Thomas M: *Psychiatric Mental Health Nursing: Application of the Nursing Process*. Philadelphia: J.B. Lippincott, 1990.

STRAUSS J: Mediating processes in schizophrenia: Towards a new dynamic psychiatry. *British Journal of Psychiatry* 155(suppl.5):22–28, 1989.

Additional Readings

FRIES J, ERLICH G (eds): *Prognosis, Contemporary Outcomes of Disease*. Bowie, MD: The Charles Press, 1981.

KATON W, KLEINMEN A: A biopsychosocial approach to surgical evaluation and outcome. *Western Journal of Medicine* 33:9–14, 1980.

MCELVEEN-HOEHN P: The cooperation model for care in health and illness. In Chaska N (ed): *The Nursing Profession*, Vol 2. New York: McGraw-Hill, 1982.

RAHE R: Subject's recent life changes and their near future illness reports. *Annals of Clinical Research* 4:250–265, 1972.

5

Decision Making in Nursing Treatment Planning

Diagnostic and prognostic judgments are not ends in themselves, only steps, but crucial steps toward determining what actions to take—nursing treatment.

What Is Nursing Treatment?

Nursing treatment is any action or behavior undertaken by the nurse in the professional role in order to affect:

1. The patient's or family's responses to: a) health-related experiences and b) capacities to manage daily living as it is affected by health status and health-related experiences.
2. The situation within which this health-related experience is occurring and external factors affecting the patient's and family's health status and responses.

Nursing treatment may be planned in advance and then carried out. However, many times it is more spontaneous and may seem unplanned. It can be carried out by the nurse who planned the care or delegated to others.

Nursing treatment is based on judgments[1] (made with or without awareness) about the patient's or family's status or situation. These judgments may have been formalized into diagnostic and prognostic statements or may be just impressions. However, nursing treatment is based on some level of clinical judgment about the patient's or family's status and situation.

Some nurses limit their definition of nursing treatment to those actions actually documented on a care plan or patient record. Nursing treatment as described in this chapter, encompasses much more than that. At present, a very small proportion of nursing treatment given to patients and families is actually written down either before or after it has occurred. Many nurses provide the bulk of their nursing treatment without even being aware that they are treating patients and their situations. For example:

A frail 80-year-old woman who was admitted to the nursing home from her own home two days ago is sitting in a wheelchair in the hallway, alone. She is cognitively alert and her sight and hearing are relatively intact.

A nurse walks by en route to bringing a medication to another resident. She stops, faces the resident, touches her hand and says, "You're looking very pretty in your blue dress today, Mrs. Talbot," and then continues on her original errand.

[1]A nursing judgment is a decision or conclusion derived from data from or about patients and their situations. See also Chapter 1, p. 3.

This nurse "treated" the resident by providing the sensory input of touch, opportunity for eye contact and sound, and potentially contributed to the resident's self-esteem.

In a neonatal intensive care unit, one nurse consistently uses personal as well as task-oriented touch and talks to the babies when they are awake during feeding and treatments. Another nurse gives equally skilled medical, personal, and feeding care, uses only task-oriented touch and talks about, but not directly to, the infant. Both nurses are integrating nursing treatment with the medical care. The first nurse's care contributes to the infant's well-being. The second nurse's care may contribute to failure-to-thrive syndrome.

Because the domain for nursing treatment involves human responses to health-related experiences, the occasions for nursing treatment are much less circumscribed than those of medicine. Any nursing contact is part of the patient's and family's health-related experience and therefore is an occasion for nursing treatment. Failure to treat or deciding not to carry out an action are forms of treatment.
See *Exercise Set 1* for activities to explore the nature of nursing treatment.

Foundations for Nursing Treatment Decisions

Nursing treatment is grounded in both clinical knowledge and patient data. It is based on:

- The identified status and situation of the recipient.
- Knowledge about the variables involved in the response or situation, their linkages and dynamics.
- A judgment about the likely course of events and outcome of the diagnosed problem based on data about the strengths and deficits in the situation and knowledge about usual patterns in such problem areas—a prognosis
- Any additional relevant data about requirements in the person's daily living and the functional capacities and external resources needed and available to meet those requirements.
- Knowledge about the nursing treatment options available and the way in which specific interventions are predicted to affect underlying mechanisms in the situation, both desired effects and possible side effects.

Identified Status and Situation

The identified status or situation of the person being treated is the initial focus in determining what is to be treated. Obviously, the more specific the focus is, the more specific the treatment can be.

Treatment based on a formalized diagnosis (whether documented or in the nurse's thoughts), can address the identified problem area, related factors, or response. For example:

The diagnosis is: Recent social isolation R/T stroke-caused dysphagia L/T anger and depression.

Treating the related factors. If the dysphagia is of a type that can be rehabilitated, treatment is directed toward teaching the patient how to gain insight into the problem and how to swallow with neuromuscular deficits (Axelsson, 1988; Heimlich, 1983; Ozuna, 1991, pp. 1165–1166). If treatment of the dysphagia is successful, social isolation and the responses of anger and depression may also be resolved.

Treating the problem area. If the dysphagia is of a type that cannot be rehabilitated, then treatment could be directed toward helping the patient to develop strategies for managing social situations in the presence of dysphagia.

Treating the response. If the patient is unable or unwilling to learn new social skills surrounding the dysphagia, if people with whom he would like to socialize are unwilling to accept him with his disability, and if his social situation remains unsatisfactory, treatment would be directed toward helping him find compensatory situations and managing anger and depression as effectively as possible.

See **Exercise Set 2-1** for activities addressing treatment of different parts of the nursing diagnosis.

It is difficult to write about the less conscious nursing impressions that form a basis for nursing treatment, since putting them into words automatically makes them a conscious thought. However, one might think of situations where a nurse had some impressions and acted on them. For example:

A child whose physiological status is obviously and inevitably deteriorating is trying to control all other aspects of her life and the people around her, including the nursing staff. One nurse, at some level of awareness, senses the child's underlying anxiety and search for control. Without putting vague impressions into words, this nurse's intuitive nursing actions are to support hope, legitimize the child's feelings, help the child to communicate her needs in effective ways and, as much as possible, create opportunities for taking control in daily living.

Another nurse, who does not sense the anxiety being manifested in controlling behavior, might seek to reduce or reject the controlling behavior.

Whether nurses' perceptions of a situation are intuitive impressions or formalized into a diagnostic format, they form the focus and basis for treatment. And, whatever the level of awareness, their focus and accuracy are initial factors in the effectiveness of the treatment. For example, suppose nurses in the cases above:

Made an erroneous judgment that a treatable dysphagia could not respond to treatment and instead focused on adapting to daily living with a feeding tube.

Did not sense the child's anxiety but felt the child was manipulative and difficult.

Based on different diagnoses or impressions, it is obvious that the treatment for each patient would be quite different. Wrong nursing diagnoses result in wrong nursing treatment.

Some nurses have felt that nursing diagnoses and judgments are innocuous. That is not true. They are the basis for nursing actions, and those actions or the failure to take action affect the well-being of patients and their families. If the diagnosis or impression is incorrect, nursing action is likely to be, at the least, inappropriate and, at the worst, harmful.

See *Exercise Set 2-2* for activities exploring nursing treatment given without awareness.

Knowledge About Underlying Dynamics

Nursing treatment is focused by diagnosis or judgment, but it evolves on the basis of knowing what variables are involved and how they interact, in other words, the **underlying dynamics** or **underlying mechanisms.**

Physiology, Pathophysiology, and Psychopathology

Some underlying mechanisms involved in understanding the dynamics of nursing problems concern physiology, pathophysiology, or psychopathology as these affect functional capacities. Figure 5-1 illustrates these relationships when a patient has the potential for or is experiencing pathology and its medical treatment. For example:

Dyspnea associated with an acute lower respiratory infection in a normally healthy person is of limited duration, while that in a person with end-stage respiratory or cardiac disease is ongoing and progressive (Gold, 1983). Dyspnea associated with advancing cancer shows a typical pattern of discrete episodes with slow onset, a lengthy plateau and a gradual decrease in the dyspnea (Brown et al., 1986). With cancer progression, the episodes recur more frequently until there is little or no interval between them. Nursing treatment of helping individuals to manage daily living with different kinds of dyspnea is not going to be the same, but will be based on how the pathophysiology affects their functional capacities.

Episodes of hostile, combative behavior in individuals with psychopathology (e.g., Alzheimer's disease) show a typical pattern of prodromal manifestations, escalation, peaking, and de-escalation (Crandall, 1993). Nursing treatment at each of these phases is different.

Anxiety occurs at four different levels (Peplau, 1963; Whitley, 1991). At higher levels stimuli overwhelm the capacity of the reticular activating system, and

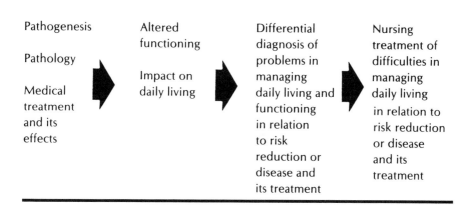

Pathogenesis

Pathology

Medical
treatment
and its
effects

Altered
functioning

Impact on
daily living

Differential
diagnosis of
problems in
managing
daily living and
functioning
in relation
to risk
reduction or
disease and
its treatment

Nursing
treatment of
difficulties in
managing
daily living
in relation to
risk reduction
or disease
and its
treatment

FIGURE 5-1 Nursing's Knowledge Base for Treatment Planning. Adapted from Carnevali D, Reiner A: *The Cancer Experience: Nursing Diagnosis and Management.* Philadelphia: J.B. Lippincott, 1990. p. 3.

cortical arousal is high, resulting in sensory overload (Lee, 1991, p. 80). Nursing treatment at each level varies (Carpenito, 1989, pp. 133–134).

See *Exercise Set 2-3* for activities on variations in nursing treatment associated with common symptoms but different underlying pathology.

Medical Activities and Their Effects

Medical diagnostic and treatment activities affect the pathology and pathophysiology they are intended to diagnose, prevent or, treat. It is important to note that they also affect other aspects of patient response and the situation of the patient, family members, or caregivers. Fear and anxiety associated with anticipation of tests and treatment can disrupt usual functioning. Travel for frequent treatments that must be performed in an institutional setting can create discomfort, expense, and disruption of other activities. Time and discomfort associated with carrying out treatments, even in the home, disrupt normal routines and perhaps make other aspects of daily living difficult if not impossible. For example:

> Some treatments associated with respiratory hygiene can occupy hours of each day for a person with advanced chronic obstructive pulmonary disease (COPD). Constant use of oxygen creates new demands and limitations on mobility, shopping, and travel (Lareau, 1993).

Some treatments result in increased functional capacities—greater strength and endurance, freedom from pain and other symptoms. Other treatments produce side effects that create their own problems. For example:

- Hair loss associated with chemotherapy.
- Impotence as a side effect of certain medications.
- Modification of perception associated with psychoactive drugs.
- Disfigurement and dysfunction associated with some surgery.

These effects can vary in magnitude and duration and thus affect the nature of nursing treatment needed to assist the patient and caregivers in managing their daily lives.

See *Exercise Set 2-4* for activities on impact of medical activities on need for nursing treatment.

Other Variables Internal and External to the Person

Nursing treatment can be concerned with many types of responses that may have little to do with pathology. Examples of these include:

- Chronologic age-associated physical and cognitive status.
- Type and level of education.
- Command of the language used by care providers.
- Previous life experiences that affect current attitudes, values and responses in the health situation.
- Earlier approaches to life challenges.
- Usual pessimism or optimism.
- Feelings about independence or dependence.
- Comfort in relating to others.
- Developmental task achievement or those yet to be achieved.

Each of these are variables that can affect individualized nursing treatment of diagnosed areas.

Other probable variables include requirements in daily living, such as activities, events, role responsibilities, self-expectations, environment, values and beliefs (Carnevali, 1988; 1990). The patient's and family's external resources also tend to be important variables. These include:

- *Architecture of housing:* stairs, distances, location of bathroom, cooking facilities, laundry facilities, space for privacy and for socialization, dormitory-type architecture in shelters for the homeless (beds close together, enhancing exposure to organisms, and threats to personal safety).
- *Communication:* availability of telephone, emergency number, e.g., 911.
- *Financial resources:* income, health insurance, obligations, debts, and money for health-related services, supplies, equipment.
- *Housing:* availability of housing, security, furnishings, amenities.
- *Neighborhood:* character, safety, facilities, density of people, distances, terrain.
- *People:* personal networks of family and friends who are or are not available to help; individuals or groups who are a threat to personal well-being.
- *Pets:* household animals, birds, or fish available for contact or as a responsibility.

- *Services:* level of availability and usability of services of health care systems, governmental and social services from any source.
- *Supplies and equipment:* availability of health-related supplies and equipment through commercial or volunteer organizations.
- *Technology:* availability of needed and desired health care technology; availability of possibly undesired technology.
- *Transportation:* nature and availability of usable private or public transportation, e.g., wheelchair or limited mobility access to buses, private vehicles the person can get into and out of, specialized transportation, e.g., the "Buddy and Bucket Brigade" (volunteers with appropriate equipment and supplies who drive patients to and from cancer treatments where the treatment side effect is nausea and vomiting). (Carnevali and Reiner, 1990; Carnevali, 1993)

See *Exercise Set 2-5* for activities on identification of patient data needed for treatment decisions.

Prognosis

Another area of consideration in planning treatment is that of the prognosis for the situation. This involves knowledge about patterns of course of events and outcomes and prognostic variables. It also involves data on prognostic variables from the patient's situation as described in Chapter 4.

See *Exercise Set 2-6* for activities identifying the influence of prognosis on treatment decisions.

Additional Data

Treatment decisions often require patient data that are different from those collected in the initial assessment. Data needed for treatment decisions also go beyond those involved in the diagnosis.

Strengths and Adequacy of External Resources

Nursing treatment is instituted because the patient or family are unable to manage the demands of the situation without nursing help. However, no patient or family is totally without strengths. A seriously ill person may have only the will to live, but that is a strength that can be fostered. External resources may be minimal but there are usually some, and these can be used and nurtured in nursing treatment. Activities, events, demands, and environments in daily living usually present both strengths and challenges. Values and beliefs also can create either strengths or deficits in living with the health situation.

Nursing treatment compensates for functional deficits, for inadequate or inappropriate resources, and seeks to modify requirements in daily living that cannot be met. However, nursing treatment is built on the patient's or family members' strengths, the positive elements in daily living and the external resources that are available and usable. Therefore, data on relevant positive elements in the situation are essential to effective treatment planning.

Status of Others Who Share the Patient's Health Experiences

Very few individuals, whether engaged in a health promotion experience or an illness experience, go through that experience alone. Usually others share the daily living and health-related experiences with the person. Often their health status, their values and priorities affect the patient and the situation; and their participation can be crucial to the well-being of the patient. For example:

> Suppose an individual is trying to lose weight. The food preparer loves to cook, believes that feeding is loving, and that eating the prepared food indicates that love is returned. The food preparer's beliefs and behavior can make the challenge of weight reduction exceedingly difficult.

> A child is being sent home from the hospital on a ventilator. The mother is a single parent with several other children. Her physical and mental status will be crucial to her ability to provide adequate physical and emotional care to the patient and siblings.

> A man is in a coronary care unit after having suffered a coronary infarct. His wife is anxiously hovering about and speaking in a loud frantic voice. The patient exhibits greater cardiac abnormalities when she is allowed into the unit.

> A woman in her forties is undergoing pelvic irradiation. She and her husband have had an active and satisfying sexual relationship and wish to continue. Both will need to learn modifications that can enable each of them to continue to be satisfied with their sexuality (Carnevali and Reiner, 1990).

> A woman is terminally ill with cancer. Her husband has not accepted her dying and keeps begging her to hold on, that perhaps a cure will come. She struggles to remain alive for him in spite of increasing suffering.

In each of these instances, it will not be enough to treat the patient. Some form of treatment, either through the patient or with the significant other(s), will be needed.

Knowledge About Nursing Treatment Options

In order to make treatment decisions, one must know what treatment options are available within the discipline, what human responses or elements of the situation they can affect, and what their effects and side effects are. This includes not only discipline-specific treatment modalities in general but also specific treatment protocols modifications that are possible for particular diagnoses and individualizing.

Nursing's Discipline-specific Treatment Modalities

Certain treatment modalities are associated with each health care discipline (Bulecheck and McCloskey, 1985). Medicine includes such treatment options as biological and chemical substances (medications), surgery, radiation, physiotherapy, prostheses, electrical and magnetic forces, mechanical devices, computers, psychotherapy, gene therapy. Nursing also has modalities that are options in treatment decisions. The following list includes some of them:

- Providing physical assistance with activities and treatments that will supplement, complement, or substitute for the person's deficits.
- Altering or helping the patient to alter the physical, microbial or sensory environment for safety, comfort, or efficiency.
- Providing experiences to permit insight, learning, or skills.
- Providing a safe environment in which to practice skills or rehearse behaviors.
- Providing opportunities to examine values, attitudes, goals, and expectations associated with the health situation.
- Assisting the person to reframe a situation to gain a different perspective.
- Providing knowledge or sources of knowledge appropriate to a person's ability to understand and offered at a time when the person is able to participate in learning.
- Helping the person to find ways of applying knowledge to relevant areas of daily living.
- Giving assistance or support in planning health-related daily living.
- Developing contracts as a means of supporting the person's commitment to undertake and maintain selected activities or behaviors.
- Providing expertise and support in dealing/negotiating with health care bureaucracies or personnel.
- Making contacts with other external resources or expediting their use.
- Supporting maintenance of external resources.
- Helping to develop and rehearse a repertoire of "scripts" or behaviors for dealing with predicted difficult interactions or situations.
- Arranging for or suggesting strategies for effective respite from demands of daily living for patient, primary caregiver, or family members.
- Legitimizing feelings and experiences generated by health-related situations and offering strategies for gaining self/others' acceptance of those responses.
- Providing or assisting in arranging sensory stimulation that is meaningful and of an appropriate magnitude and amount.
- Scheduling or assisting in planning schedules for activities or events commensurate with the current or predicted functional capacities.
- Finding ways to incorporate preferred patterns and valued activities into daily living when health status or health care activities make this difficult.
- Providing a personal presence, genuinely being there, touching.
- Recommending and supporting strategies for managing painful or stressful experiences.
- Assisting patients/family members in learning new role behaviors, relationships

and role expectations associated with the health experience. (Carnevali, 1992; Carnevali and Reiner, 1990)

Nursing textbooks identify nursing treatments that have been found to be effective in dealing with diagnosed phenomena or situations. There are standard care plans, nursing protocols or care standards that identify general treatments. These contribute to the knowledge base needed about treatment options. In addition, clinical practice hones, refines, and adds to the treatments a nurse is prepared to offer; variations and individualizing modifications are regularly added.

See *Exercise Set 3-1* for activities to extrapolate nursing treatment modalities from nursing activities.

Specific Treatment for Variations in a Phenomenon

Treatment guidelines often are offered for a general category of phenomena. However, it is not enough to utilize general treatment when specific treatment is needed. For example: management of daily living with hallucinations in general includes four major forms of treatment:

1. Monitoring the content of hallucinations.
2. Safety and protective measures.
3. Teaching voice dismissal.
4. Interaction with others (Thomas and Sanger, 1989).

In one study, hallucinatory patterns were found to have associated diagnostic clusters (ADC).

1. **Command-auditory:** ADC—suicide potential, potential for violence to others, anxiety.
2. **Accusatory/derogatory-auditory** (and often threatening visual hallucinations): ADC—persecutory delusions, potential for violence toward others, social isolation, self-care deficits.
3. **Multisensory** with diffuse difficulties in thinking and acting: ADC—alterations in thought processes, bizarre behavior, personal identity disturbance.
4. **Chronic** hallucinations (usually auditory but may involve other senses): ADC— social isolation, difficulty in structuring time.
5. **Iatrogenic** hallucinations (usually visual) due to medication side effects: ADC— medication toxicity, anxiety. (Thomas and Sanger, 1989).

These diagnostic clusters resulted in treatment recommendations in which some of the general treatments were appropriate, some needed modifications, and others were contraindicated as shown below.

Type of hallucination	Treatment[2]
Command-auditory hallucinations diagnostic cluster	1. Monitor content of hallucinations— **assess ongoing risks.**

[2]Note that modifications of the standard treatment appear in boldface type.

2. Safety measures—**close observation or suicide precautions. Protection of others.**
3. Teach voice dismissal (**after the acute stage**).
4. Interaction with others **unless anxiety level is high.**

Accusatory derogatory hallucinations diagnostic cluster

1. Monitor content of hallucinations—**assess ongoing risks.**
2. Safety measures—**close observation or suicide precautions. Protection of others.**
3. Teach voice dismissal (**after the acute stage**).
4. **Limit** interaction with others to avoid increase in hallucinations and potential for violence. **Only peripheral involvement in groups.**

Multisensory with diffuse difficulties in thinking and acting diagnostic cluster

1. Focus on content of hallucinations is **counterproductive. Encourage more appropriate communication.**
2. Safety measures—**protect the patient because of inability for self-care.**
3. Teach voice dismissal (**after the acute stage**).
4. **Selective** interaction with others **limited to one or a very few others** to prevent patient being overwhelmed.

Chronic hallucinations diagnostic cluster

1. **Assess meaning of hallucinations** (irritating/comforting) **instead of focusing on content.**
2. Safety measures **usually not needed.**
3. Teach voice dismissal—**very important,** particularly if voices are irritating.
4. **Increased** interaction with others **important** since this tends to reduce hallucinations and decrease social isolation.

Iatrogenic-visual hallucination diagnostic cluster

1. Monitoring content of hallucinations **not relevant.**

2. Safety measures: **protect patient** because of limitations on self-care.
3. Teaching voice dismissal **inappropriate.**
4. **Limit** interaction with others to **frequent contact with a few consistent individuals. Limit outside stimuli.**
(Thomas and Sanger, 1989)

It can be seen that, even within the same phenomenon (hallucinations), standard nursing interventions may need to be modified, emphasized, or avoided depending on the kind of hallucinatory experience and the associated diagnostic cluster.

See *Exercise Set 3-2* for activities to consider variations on nursing treatment related to variations within a nursing diagnostic category.

Specific Treatment for Levels or Stages in a Phenomenon

Not only is treatment made specific for variations in a particular phenomenon, it is also varied for different levels or stages within a phenomenon.

Anxiety is a human response that has been identified as having different gradations of severity ranging from mild to panic. As shown in Figure 5-2, breadth and clarity of perception and level of attention and capacity for learning or problem solving vary markedly. These variations affect nursing treatment that involves learning, problem solving and ability to perceive external stimuli. Teaching and assistance with problem solving as nursing treatments are possible and may even be enhanced in mild levels of anxiety but inappropriate and possibly harmful at higher levels. Limiting external stimuli is less a concern at the lower levels but becomes a high priority for nursing treatment at higher levels.

Just as some phenomena are described in terms of levels, others are considered in terms of phases or stages. Grief work and adaptation to chronic illness are examples of phenomena that are characterized as having several possible phases. Treatment options that are ideal at one phase would be highly inappropriate during another.

See *Exercise Set 3-3* for activities to explore variations in treatment linked to levels of severity within a nursing diagnosis.

Nursing treatment decisions then are based on a solid foundation of knowledge about general treatment options available and specific ones associated with the particular phenomenon or situation being treated. This is the knowledge for standard acceptable treatment. However, to individualize care so that it fits with a particular patient situation, treatment decisions need to be derived from additional data on requirements in daily living and the patient's current and predicted strengths and resources as well as deficits. In addition, treatment consideration needs to be given to those who closely share the patient's health-related experiences and whose daily living and functioning affect patient outcomes.

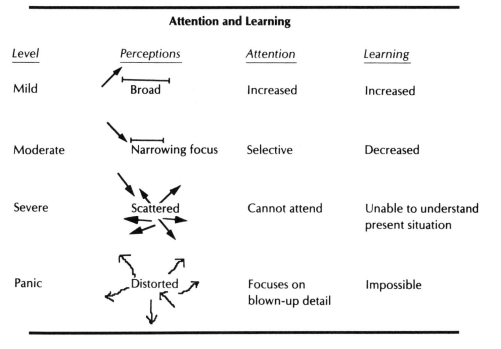

FIGURE 5-2   Characteristics of Levels of Anxiety. Adapted from Figure 9-1 in Carnevali D: *Sykepleieplanlegging*. Oslo: Gyldendal Norsk Forlag, 1992

Models for Decision Making

Two models have been used to analyze decision making for treatment in nursing. *Decision analysis* considers a rational, logical approach to choosing between mutually exclusive options. *Opportunistic planning* examines strategies that can be used to seek promising options as they occur rather than consistently moving through a systematic pattern.

Decision Analysis Model

Decision analysis focuses on what decision is to be made rather than the process for making it. However, as one engages in formalized steps of decision analysis, treatment options and patient data tend to replicate the processes of other rational approaches to treatment decisions. One of the differences is the use of quantification and mathematical operations to arrive at the decision. The goal is to efficiently utilize available information and knowledge in order to arrive at a decision that fits with both preferences and judgment (Raiffa, 1968).

Decision analysis provides a structure and a series of steps for choosing a treatment option from among mutually exclusive possibilities.[3] It involves four steps:

1. Structure and fill in a decision-flow diagram incorporating information about *decision forks*—options or choices the decision maker has (designated as squares), *chance forks*—factors over which the decision maker has no control (designated as circles) and *possible outcomes* at the distal tip of each branch. The decision flow diagram is illustrated in Figure 5-3.

2. Assign a *value score (v)* to each possible outcome. This can be done as a two-step operation by first ranking them in order of preference and then assigning an arbitrary number to each ranking. The range for the value numbers is the decision maker's choice. One could, for example, choose a range of 0 to 100 or -10 to $+10$, etc. Using these two ranges as examples, total success of the treatment would be scored as a 100 or a $+10$, the worst outcome would receive a 0 or a -10. Those that reflect varying degrees of positive or negative outcomes could be assigned values in between.

3. Make a mathematical judgment about the *likelihood or probability (p) that a chance response or event will occur*. These judgments may be objective—based on information about previous frequency of occurrence, or subjective—based on one's personal experience or beliefs about the frequency of occurrence. The numbers assigned must add up to 1.0 for each fork. So, if there is a 50–50 chance that either of the possibilities would occur, the p value would be 0.5 for each of them, adding up to 1.0 for the two. The assigned p value is written on each branch of the fork.

4. Do the following mathematical calculations to arrive at the decision that has the highest value:
   - Multiply the probability score *(p)* by the assigned value score *(v)* for each chance fork *(p × v)*, e.g., a response has a 0.5 chance of occurring and is valued at 7. *(p × v = 3.5)*.
   - Repeat this process for each of the distal forks.
   - Add the $p × v$ *(pv)* for each set of distal forks.
   - Place the sum in the oval where the forks join (designated b on Figure 5-3).
   - Add the 2 numbers at the pairs of b's. Place this number at the oval above the options designated a on Figure 5-3.
   - The option with the highest number is the one judged to be the best or the most preferred one.

One area where decision analysis can be useful in nursing is that of helping patients or families to make informed decisions or engage in informed consent about treatment, e.g., to put an ailing, disoriented, aged parent on kidney dialysis (Hoffart, 1993); to seek a "Do Not Resuscitate" injunction; to decide whether to have radical surgery for prostatic cancer when there is a coexisting cardiac condition that may

---

[3]In mutually exclusive possibilities, the making of one choice eliminates the possibility of making another. For example, if one is deciding between driving the car to the store or walking, the choice of one eliminates the other. One cannot simultaneously drive the car and walk to the store.

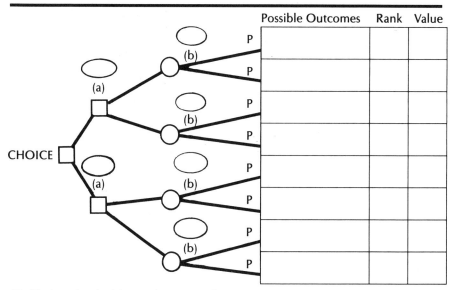

	Possible Outcomes	Rank	Value
P			
P			
P			
P			
P			
P			
P			
P			

☐ Choices the decision maker can make
○ Chance events
P   Objective or subjective probability the event will occur
⬭ Sum of (probability x value) of each fork

FIGURE 5-3   Decision Analysis Tree

prove terminal before the cancer; to share information such as one's history of cancer or HIV positive status; or to take a certain action (leaving an institution against medical advice). These are decisions that are mutually exclusive (at least for a time) and therefore lend themselves to decision analysis. Further, the activity of decision analysis offers an opportunity for consideration of both rational and value-laden aspects of the choice. Note that research has shown that the way in which the risks and benefits of options are worded can seriously affect the choices made (Tversky and Kahneman, 1981).

Limitations of Application in Nursing

There are certain limitations in the application of decision analysis to nursing treatment decisions. Nursing treatment options are frequently not "either–or" but can be taken together. Using clusters of treatment as mutually exclusive options increases the complexity of decision analysis. Nursing outcomes may be difficult to quantify, and the outcomes tend not be stable or final.

Using a subjective approach in assigning probability scores can be affected by recent experiences and dramatic previous events rather than a broader look at patterns of frequencies.

Decision analysis takes time. Many decisions about nursing treatment cannot be predicted and actions must be taken quickly. Decision analysis is therefore not useful for many nursing treatment decisions.

Uses of Decision Analysis in Nursing

When decision analysis can be used in nursing, it can bring benefits to both the nurse and the person being treated.

For nurses, the process and structure forces them to be specific about mutually exclusive options, consider the most productive treatments and likely outcomes for each, and finally, to separate probabilities from values (Corcoran, 1986a). Nurses can gain insight about limitations on their control over outcomes because of intervening variables and also can begin to look at outcome frequencies associated with particular nursing therapies.

If nurses involve those who are to receive treatment in the decision making process, there is an opportunity for patients and families to gain new insights into possibilities, options, and the values they hold. In the end this could result in greater commitment to the eventual decision.

Because it is time consuming, decision analysis may find a place in clinical practice only with complex or recurrent problems. In either of these instances, costs in time and energy may be balanced by satisfaction that the choice of action has been considered fully. For recurrent problems, benefits may come in more effective decision making for subsequent cases based on better data collection and more rapid consideration of probabilities and values that will vary with individual patient situations.

See *Exercise Set 4-1* for activities in use of decision analysis protocols and forms.

Opportunistic Versus Systematic Approaches in Treatment Decisions

Planning treatment is at least as complex a cognitive task as that of making the diagnosis. While the focus has been determined by that diagnosis, there are many other variables affecting treatment decisions. Task complexity has been found to influence the way information is processed (Payne, 1982). Certainly, the memory limitations that applied in the diagnostic reasoning process are present as well in making treatment decisions.

One approach to planning for treatment has been labeled "opportunistic planning" (Hayes-Roth and Hayes-Roth, 1979; Corcoran, 1986b). Its name comes from the belief that, in complex planning, individuals pursue whatever leads seem currently promising or opportune without systematically reviewing all possible options. For example:

Several nurses are eating in the hospital cafeteria. At a nearby table next to a glass partition, they see a man begin to make violent jerking movements, his body tips toward the glass partition and his head bangs against it. His mouth is full of food. He appears to have lost consciousness. The nurse from the neurology unit moves over to his side quickly, gets help in laying him on his side on the floor, sweeps out the food in his mouth and slips a napkin into the side of the mouth, then places a jacket under his head until the involuntary movement quiets.

Engaging in opportunistic decision making, the nurse focused on priorities of avoiding cuts to his head from broken glass and maintaining an airway in a person who had been eating, was unconscious, and having a grand mal seizure.

Opportunistic planning can proceed in a seemingly disorderly multidirectional manner as the planner considers useful approaches. Experienced clinicians have been found to ask fewer questions, collect less data, and focus on those areas that are most likely to yield maximum information (Kleinmutz, 1968). Expert nurses making decisions about weaning patients from ventilators recognized when to retain and when to abandon lines of reasoning (Narayan, 1990). This contrasts with the approach of moving systematically through all parts of a pre-set routine in one's thinking.

Creators of the model acknowledge that opportunistic planning makes greater demands on memory capacity. Research analyzing novice and expert behavior planning treatment in *simulated patient situations* found that nurses using opportunistic thinking lost some of the earlier options they had considered. They identified more options than they could then later recall when it was time to make their treatment decisions (Corcoran, 1986b). In practice, expert nurses in familiar situations may well primarily consider those actions that they have found to be therapeutic (Narayan, 1990). Expert nurses were found to consistently use the opportunistic model in the most complex cases and the systematic approach in the least complex cases (Corcoran, 1986b).

Different kinds of problem solving (treatment) require different types of cognitive strategies (McGuire, 1985). Early studies of medical students' management of patient problems showed that they tended to use the same strategy in all types of patient situations, and that this pattern produced an inferior product (McGuire and Babbott, 1967). Adjusting strategies of decision making to task complexity is important for effective treatment.

It is suggested that opportunistic planning can result in more varied and better plans. Where cases are complex, this approach is worth consideration, provided strategies are used to cluster information or options so that the risk of losing important materials is minimized.

Opportunistic thinking can be managed by identification of *constant threads*. For example:

The nurse caring for a person with schizophrenia will need to consider that altered thought processes and perceptions and difficulty in structuring time will be constant threads in planning treatment to manage requirements of daily living such as eating, sleeping, relating, elimination, going to work or school.

Identification and use of the constant thread in a situation can economize on working memory space.

Opportunistic thinking can also be managed by *grouping problems and integrating treatment*. For example:

> To some extent, problems of eating, fluid intake, and elimination can be grouped in treatment planning. Further, if socialization is a concern, it too could be integrated into the activity of eating. Where pain interferes with eating, it would also need to be integrated.

Clustering and integration of a variety of treatment areas is not only economical in opportunistic thinking, it is critical to effective nursing treatment.

See *Exercise 4-2* for activities using opportunistic thinking in treatment decisions.

Elements of the Process for Making Treatment Decisions in Nursing

Just as there were recognizable elements in the process of arriving at diagnostic and prognostic judgments, there are elements in making decisions about treatment. Essentially the cognitive processes and use of memory is the same; however, different content elements are involved.

The same memory limitations and constraints that characterized thinking strategies in the process of making clinical judgments described in earlier chapters apply here as well. Planning for almost any form of individualized nursing treatment is a complex task if it is well done. The skill comes in being able to retain the realistic and necessary complexity within the 5–9 chunks of working memory capacity. Maintaining an awareness that one must cluster knowledge and data in order to be able to create individualized nursing treatment may help nurses to develop organization patterns and strategies that minimize loss of necessary information.

Areas for decision making involved in treatment planning are discussed in the next section. As with diagnostic reasoning, cognitive processes involved in these decisions may occur at different levels of awareness. Treatment decisions are sometimes made almost instantaneously, without conscious thought. At other times they are approached over longer periods of time. In this chapter all elements of decision making are necessarily spelled out discretely and described in some detail. In the real world of clinical practice, some elements may be skipped or blended. It is hoped that by describing these elements fully, readers can develop cognitive strategies and patterns resulting in more individualized and effective nursing treatment.

Basic decisions and actions needed to plan individualized nursing treatment are outlined in Display 5-1.

DISPLAY 5-1
OVERVIEW OF ELEMENTS OF THE PROCESS FOR MAKING
TREATMENT DECISIONS IN NURSING.

Determine what is to be treated.

Determine the outcome to be achieved by the treatment.

Consider time lines for the treatment.

Consider the treatment options that could achieve the intended outcome.

Obtain or review data on strengths or deficits in the situation that must be integrated into treatment decisions.

Consult with the recipient of the treatment about the treatment.

Decide on the overall treatment plan and specific elements.

Decide who is to be involved in implementation.

Decide how to communicate the treatment activities to any others who will be involved in implementation.

Decision on What Is To Be Treated

The diagnosis provides guidelines for what is to be treated. However, within the diagnosis there are several potential areas for treatment. One may treat the problem, the related factors, or the response as described earlier in the chapter. It is important to decide which aspect(s) are to be targeted. Different actions may need to be prescribed for each area if more than one is to receive treatment. For example:

A man is being treated for lung cancer with radiation of the mediastinum and is suffering from esophagitis with swelling and pain. He has difficulty eating and is restricting his food to one variety of thin creamed soup. The wife is a good cook and has been trying unsuccessfully to get her husband to eat some other liquid-soft foods as well. He refuses and she is upset. Her distress and her efforts to change his eating patterns are distressing the husband. (The diagnosis focuses on the wife.)

Frustration with monotony of food preparation R/T husband's resistance to varying his limited diet 2° radiation esophagitis L/T nagging, anger, guilt.

To treat the response one could institute immediate treatment of the feelings of anger and guilt by legitimization of those feelings and giving realistic information about the limited duration of iatrogenic esophagitis. The response of "nagging" could be addressed through consideration of alternative scripts and approaches, or reframing the situation.

To treat related factors, the nurse: 1) could consult the patient about the variety of cream soups he would be willing to try and also some comparably textured foods that might be easy to swallow and retain, 2) check on use of an effective level of analgesics 30–45 minutes prior to eating.

To treat frustration with the monotony, one could help the wife take care of her own eating, legitimizing preparation of foods that she likes, and consider ways of serving the limited foods in ways that create variety and use her creative talent.

Each area of the diagnosis targeted for treatment requires a different approach.

It is important to determine which of the elements lend themselves to nursing treatment and which should or can be treated first. The diagnosis is a gestalt in creating the focus for treatment but its parts need to be considered in terms of specific treatment decisions.

Decision on the Outcomes Treatments Are Intended to Achieve

Treatment will vary with a given diagnosis depending on the outcomes to be achieved. To make this decision one needs to consider the prognostic data and prognosis.

Prognosis and Prognostic Data

Ideally a prognosis has been considered in conjunction with the diagnosis. To plan treatment one needs to consider not only the prognosis but the supporting prognostic data. Often these data will play an important role in the actual treatments themselves. Prognostic data usually incorporate information about strengths and deficits in functional capacities, external resources, and earlier/current/future patterns of daily living and managing of health-related challenges. These strengths or deficits would be integrated into the treatment.

Choice of Prognostic Outcomes

In Chapter 4 several prognostic possibilities were described. These included prevention/delay/minimization of a potential problem, resolution of a problem, stabilization of a fluctuating situation that cannot be resolved, and palliation or support in a situation that cannot be resolved and appears to be inevitably deteriorating.

Again, treatment will be different for different prognostic outcomes. A crucial step in making decisions about treatment is that of determining what realistic outcome the treatment is intended to achieve.

Predicted Course of Events

The predicted course of events also affects treatment. Therefore, it is important to consider the trajectory of events as this may affect treatment. (See Chapter 4 for examples of trajectory.)

Consideration of Time Lines for the Treatment

Decisions about the predicted course of events lead to consideration about the length of time treatment will need to be continued. For example:

Dx: Knowledge and skill deficit R/T postoperative activities 2° cervical laminectomy L/T risk of complications.

Time lines for treatment will be the preoperative period, when initial teaching and rehearsal of skills will be undertaken, and the postoperative period, when activities will be important to minimize complications—probably a matter of days.

Dx: Knowledge and skill deficit in managing daily living with insulin dependent diabetes R/T newly diagnosed status L/T risk of unstable blood sugar and diabetic complications.

Time lines for treatment will be long. There may be an additional diagnosis associated with a prolonged shock or denial stage in adaptation to the diagnosis and changed body status. Knowledge and skills need to be learned at a level where prodromal symptoms are recognized and where monitoring and treatment can be integrated into daily living under wide-ranging circumstances in ways that are satisfying. The desired outcomes are complex. Nursing treatment is planned for a duration of months.

These time lines determine not only the timing of interventions but their pace and intensity. It does no good to teach postoperative behaviors after the risk period has ended. It does no good to try to teach the diabetic everything in one or two sessions. Judgment about the time line is critical to the treatment plan.

Patterns in the predicted trajectory are an important consideration. One may be able to predict times of increased need for nursing treatment and times when it may not be needed or will be needed less intensely.

Consideration of Treatment Options

Once decisions have been made or consideration given to the three elements discussed above, it is possible to consider treatment options. Here one thinks about nursing treatment modalities that are most likely to affect the identified variables in such a way as to achieve the treatment outcomes.

As in the cognitive activities associated with diagnosis and prognosis, both working and long term memory are involved in determining nursing treatment. *Working memory* contains information about the current situation. *Semantic memory* contains knowledge linked to diagnostic concepts containing the treatment options, their way of affecting the problem and the scientific rationale. *Episodic memory* contains patient instances with similar diagnoses and prognoses, treatments and responses. And ultimately, *working memory* must contain content from all of the parts of memory in order to make the final decisions.

Experienced nurses make many treatment decisions based on retrieved memory of earlier cases. Knowledge from semantic memory may well be integrated to provide a rationale for explaining or a basis for modifying treatment. Nurses with long and rich experience often have engaged in or observed more variety in nursing treatments and have observed a greater range of responses. Such nurses tend to be more adventurous—perhaps confident enough to take more risks to achieve maximum results (Corcoran, 1986c). Nurses with more limited experience, or at least limited experience with the presenting situation, tend to be more conservative, minimizing risks rather than maximizing opportunities for gains (Corcoran, 1986c). They have the semantic knowledge of what treatment is expected to do but lack the confidence bred of personal experience to know that it really happens.

In considering treatment options it is important to remember the 5–9 chunk limitations of working memory. Where possible, treatment options should be clustered and linked to avoid losing important possibilities.

Once treatment options have been retrieved into working memory, the nurse is ready to make choices among them. These choices, however, are influenced by data from the presenting situation.

Consideration of Data from the Presenting Situation

Very often, data are needed to plan treatment that were not collected in the initial nursing assessment or were not used in making the diagnosis. Nursing treatment is intended to supplement, complement and occasionally substitute for the patient's own resources. This means that there is a need for data on:

- The patient's functional strengths and developmental task achievements as well as weaknesses and developmental tasks still to be achieved.
- External resources that are available and usable as well as those creating difficulties.
- Environments that support treatment to or make it more difficult.
- Patterns in previous daily living that are pluses and supportive of the person in the current health-related situation as well as those which are nonsupportive or creating additional difficulties.
- Current daily living that is supportive as well as nonsupportive.

Nursing treatment is intended to create a balance between the requirements generated by daily living and the capacity to meet them with the goal being that health needs are achieved and quality of life is maintained at the highest level possible. Therefore it utilizes and integrates identified patient strengths and resources.

See *Exercise Set 4-3* for activities using the elements of the treatment decision process in treatment decisions.

Consultation With the Recipient of the Treatment

Much more in nursing than in medicine the patient and family are participants in the treatment plan. Although there are some recipients of nursing care who are too young or too physically or mentally dysfunctional to be able to participate in the plan of care, all patients and family members are involved in their own health care—cognitively, emotionally, and physically. For this reason it is essential that the recipient of nursing treatment be a participant in the planning at some level whenever possible.

Consultation involves listening as well as telling. Some patients and families have different ideas about how to manage health problems. There may be culturally-based differences about how health, illness, and their management are defined and addressed (Chrisman, 1991). In these situations the nurse needs to listen with respect—holding personal skepticism or disbelief in abeyance—treating the patient's or family's beliefs and wishes as neutral data.

When differences are found to exist between treatment the nurse has considered and that which is acceptable to the patient or family, negotiation is recommended (Chrisman, 1991). It is often possible to integrate the patient–family contribution with the nurses' contribution to the plan to arrive at one that is satisfactory to both.

See *Exercise Set 4-4* for activities to gain skill in interacting with patients or families in treatment decision making.

Decisions on the Treatment Plan

Final decisions on the treatment plan need to take into consideration both the gestalt and the individual elements. The plan also needs to incorporate decisions about who is to implement the plan.

The Gestalt of the Treatment Plan

Where the treatment plan encompasses more than one dimension or activity, all of the different activities need to be considered as a whole. For example:

The eating and feeding problems of the patient who had radiation-caused esophagitis cannot be adequately addressed without addressing nutrition, food appeal, food friction with esophageal surfaces, pain management, cultural factors and values related to food and eating. Both the patient and the wife, who is preparing the food and sharing the feeding-eating experience, need to be considered for treatment.

The person who has a knowledge deficit interfering with effective management of daily living with dysfunction and who also is in the shock-denial stage of adaptation cannot be adequately treated if one considers only the need for knowledge.

Substance abuse cannot be treated only physiologically. Development of strategies for managing interaction with the environment for ongoing daily living is also essential.

Very few nursing treatments can be limited to a particular task. Most often they need to take into account the broader picture of the patient's and family's situation, often including the environment for daily living in the institution or community.

See *Exercise Set 4-5* for activities to evaluate decision making using the elements of the treatment decision process.

Decisions About Specific Elements of the Treatment Plan

A treatment plan, whether medical or nursing, is made up of discrete activities. At this point in decision making about treatment, specifics become important. All that is known about

- what is to be done,
- how it is to be done,
- when and how long it is to be done,
- by whom it is to be done

is distilled from the accumulation of previous decisions and knowledge. A decision is made about specific actions to be undertaken.

Nursing Directives[4]

In order for treatment decisions to be transformed into action, they need to be translated into directives for action. These directives can take the form of:

- Thoughts that guide one's personal behavior or actions if the treatment is to be carried out by the prescriber.
- Verbalized directives (oral or written) to guide the behavior of others if the plan is to be implemented by persons other than the prescriber.

Whether it is communicated in one's thoughts, speech, or writing, directives for nursing treatment are made up of several parts as shown in Display 5-2. The clarity and precision with which each activity is specified in nursing directives will be major factors in the effectiveness with which it is implemented. One might draw an analogy with medical practice. Physicians cannot settle for a medical order that suggests a general drug category, an indefinite dosage, and vague instructions for frequency and duration of administration. Careful, correct, specific decisions are

---

[4] Sometimes known as nursing orders, nursing interventions, nursing actions, or nursing treatment plan.

DISPLAY 5-2
GUIDELINES FOR NURSING DIRECTIVES.

Verb

A command form of an active (not passive) verb specifying the exact action to be undertaken, e.g., talk, lead, listen, assist/do not assist, observe, direct, show touch/do not touch, explain, offer, request, suggest, recommend, restrict, etc. Consider carefully before using terms designating permission or control, e.g., let, allow, get-the-patient-to, as well as those that are too general to be consistently implemented, e.g., reassure, teach, support, reward, reinforce.

Adverb or Adverbial Phrase

A modifier, if needed, to tell how the action is to be taken, e.g., slowly, quickly, firmly, gently, neutrally, quietly, with enthusiasm, genuinely, with humor, seriously, at a distance of . . . inches/feet.

Content Area

A content area, if needed, e.g., type of fluids to be made available; foods or behaviors that are restricted; subject matter for conversations, teaching, discussions, feedback; part of body that is to be treated, words to use or not to use, etc., words the toddler uses and understands or using only the word(s) used by the patient-family when they talk about the cancer.

Time

Time when the activity is to be carried out. This may be a designated clock hour or may be in conjunction with:

An identified patient activity, e.g., when the patient . . . .

A nursing activity, e.g., when the nurse enters the room, before starting the medical treatment, while a nursing activity is going on.

Occurrence of a particular event or situation, e.g., before meals, during play, after school, the day before the next medical checkup.

Duration

Duration of the activity may need to be specified under certain circumstances, e.g., when the patient's endurance has a known period of tolerance, if an activity must be of a certain duration in order to be effective.

needed in all aspects of the prescription or harm can come to the patient. Nursing treatment is a professional's (or group's) decision as to actions to be taken to influence the patient and the situation. It, too, needs the same careful attention to communicating clearly the specific decisions in all aspects of the nursing prescription or harm can come to the patient.

Determination of Who Will Implement the Nursing Treatments

Individuals who will implement nursing treatment can vary. Often the nurse who planned the treatment carries out all or a portion of the specific treatments. Sometimes other nursing personnel or health care personnel implement the treatment plan. Sometimes the treatment will be effective only if a certain individual carries it out. At other times it will be effective only if all personnel are consistent in carrying out selected treatment activities.

Determinations of who will carry out the activity can be important. This decision is translated into action by communicating effectively with those who are to implement the specific nursing treatment.

Decisions on Communicating the Treatment Plan and Specific Treatment Directives to Those Who Will Implement Them

Decisions in this step involve the timing and method of communicating the treatment plan. If the treatment plan and specific directives have already been determined, the next decision is how and when to communicate the plan to others. The style and care with which this communication takes place is a factor in the attitude others will take toward the treatment plan.

Communication that will best insure that implementation of the plan will be correctly and consistently carried out may mean putting the treatment directives in writing and supplementing this by discussing it with those involved. It may mean talking individually with the person who will assume full responsibility for one or more activities. It may mean a phone call to the home health care nurse or the nurse in the nursing home, or from either of these individuals to nurses on the patient's unit in an institutional setting. Or the treatment directives may be incorporated into a transfer or discharge summary.

It does no good to carefully execute all of the steps of the diagnostic and treatment process only to have a breakdown at the point of implementation. If the patient does not receive the planned treatment, the earlier efforts are wasted. Therefore, decisions about assuring implementation are as important as any that go before them.

An added element of insurance is to follow up with any other personnel who took over responsibility for implementation. Some questions as to how the treatment was undertaken, any difficulties encountered, and patient response may insure continuation of the treatment in the way that was intended.

See *Exercise Set 5* for activities to gain skill and precision in creating nursing directives.

Summary

Decision making about nursing treatment is a complex task—probably even more complex than diagnosis. Yet the nurse is subject to the same constraints of memory limitation as were present in earlier cognitive tasks. Previous diagnostic and prognostic decisions, additional data on the presenting situation as well as knowledge and clinical experience are all combined to arrive at treatment decisions. As with all other cognitive activities involved with diagnosis and treatment in nursing, many decisions regarding personally carried out nursing treatments are made and even implemented at low levels of awareness. However, much of nursing treatment requires actions from others on a timely and consistent basis. When this is a requirement, there must be conscious decisions about creating treatment directives that clearly specify the actions to be taken with the patient or family. Finally, there are additional interpersonal factors associated with communicating about the plan with others in such a way that they integrate the planned treatment into their care of the patient.

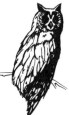

Exercises in Treatment Decision Making in Nursing

Set 1 □ The Nature of Nursing Treatment

1. Describe your ideas of what constitutes nursing treatment. Consider both planned and unplanned activities, verbal and nonverbal communication.
2. How does nursing treatment differ from delegated medical care? When you are delivering delegated medical care and nursing care, can you identify the differences? Provide some form of medical treatment to a patient and deliberately integrate nursing treatment into the interaction. Describe what you did that was the medical component and what was the nursing component.

Set 2 □ Foundations for Nursing Treatment Decisions

1. Make a nursing diagnosis that includes a specific problem area, related factors, and responses to the situation. Decide what treatment you would plan if you were to try to treat: a) the problem, b) the related factors, c) the response.
2. If possible, after encountering a patient with whom you are not familiar (one on whom you are not responsible for assessment–diagnosis):

   A. Ask your watchbird to notice any impressions you had of the patient and the situation and to give you honest, objective feedback.
   B. Try to identify any attitudes you would have toward the person, any communication patterns you would use, and behavior you would engage in the next time you encounter this patient.
   C. Repeat the activity with several patients who present different challenges to nurses. Compare your findings across patients. Do you think that your attitudes, communication, or behavior could affect the patient? Conjecture

what the effect would be. Consider how it might contribute to or detract from the patient's personal resources for managing the health experience.
D. Do you think that the casual, unplanned behavior of a nurse with a patient constitutes nursing treatment? Give a rationale for your answer.

3. Select several patients who have the same symptoms (e.g., pain, shortness of breath, fatigue, agitation) but whose pathology and pathophysiology are different. Compare the differences in pathology and pathophysiology and consider how these differences should affect the nursing (not delegated medical) treatment.

4. Select several patients. Choose from those with acute and chronic pathology. Examine the prescribed and planned medical diagnostic and treatment activities. Consider the demands that these place on the patient (emotional, comfort/discomfort, time taken by the activities, enhancement/disruption in relationships and patterns of daily living, reduced/increased need for assistance. Do the medical activities have any effect on the family, caregivers, sexual partners? Does this suggest any implications for nursing treatment of the patient or the others?

5. Select a patient. Review the sections of the chapter on "other variables internal and external to the person," pp. 114–115. Using these as a guide, gather data about the patient and situation. Think about how these findings would influence the nursing treatment you plan for the patient.

6. Using a patient on whom you have made a diagnosis and prognosis, consider how the prognosis and prognostic data affect your treatment decisions. How would your treatment plan differ if the outcomes and trajectory were different?

Set 3 □ Nursing Treatment Modalities

1. Think about the nursing activities (exclusive of delegated medical functions) in which you have engaged recently. Try to list as many types of activities as you can. Compare them to the list on pp. 117–118.

2. Consider a nursing diagnostic area in which there are variations within the diagnosis. Identify the differences in treatment needed for effectiveness with the variations.

3. Consider a nursing problem that has differing levels of severity, e.g., tiredness . . . exhaustion; mild discomfort . . . excruciating pain; indigestion . . . nausea . . . vomiting . . . retching. Identify differences in treatment needed to effectively help the person to manage the health experience.

Set 4 □ Models for Decision Making

1. A. Use Figure 5-3 as a sample and follow the instructions offered in the section on the decision analysis model, p. 122. Select a **nursing** treatment for a specific diagnosis you have made—one that has mutually exclusive options. Consider the options within each choice and the possible outcomes. Assign either known probabilities or those you subjectively believe are true. Assign

values from your perspective as a nurse. Complete the figure including the mathematical calculations.

B. What did you learn from this experience?

C. Under what circumstances would it be cost effective to use this approach to decision making?

2. A. As you plan treatment for a relatively complex patient on whom you have made a diagnosis, consider treatment options as they occur to you—as you consider levels of functioning or areas of difficulty, requirements in daily living that are compromised, external resources that are available or not/usable or not, etc. After you have decided upon the treatment, look back on the process you used. Did you find yourself overloaded with possibilities? Review your treatment plan. Do you now find that you left out important considerations or refinements because you forgot either the data or the treatment option?

B. Think back on how you could have grouped information for greater efficiency. Was there one or more constant threads that needed to be considered in all treatment decisions? Could you group several treatments under one heading? Could you integrate the treatment of several individuals (e.g., family member, caregiver, sexual partner) under one element of the treatment?

C. What did you learn from this experience?

D. Under what circumstances would you prefer to again use a similar approach to decision making? Give a rationale for your answer.

3. Use the elements outlined in Display 5-1 and the associated content as a basis for developing a treatment plan for one diagnosis on one of your patients.

4. A. Develop scripts for discussing a treatment plan you have made with the treatment recipient (patient/caregiver/family member). Select a particular patient situation and treatment plan, then role-play the interaction of talking over the treatment plan with the treatment recipient. Obtain feedback from the person playing the role of the recipient—what felt good, what was uncomfortable, what was desired but did not happen.

B. Set your watchbird to observe while you discuss this treatment plan with patients or other recipients on your unit. Critique your performance. Experiment with modifications.

5. Evaluate a treatment plan you have developed from the perspective of its quality in having taken into consideration the gestalt and having integrated the important elements effectively within nursing directives and the plan.

Set 5 □ Nursing Directives

1. A. Review the parts of the nursing directive as shown in Display 5-2. Practice writing nursing directives using these guidelines on a patient for whom you have written a diagnosis and considered a prognosis. Seek the most precise

terms possible. Make nursing directives for your own behavior and actions. Try to implement them exactly as you have prescribed in your directives. If the directive did not enable you to act as you intended, work backward from the actions and behaviors you actually did and revise your verbal directives to reflect the action or behavior and timing that was realistically needed.

B. Compare your use of these elements with your usual pattern of developing treatment plans. What are the differences? Evaluate the advantages and disadvantages of each. Could you eventually integrate these elements into your decision making process and still function quickly enough to make it practical?

C. If you decide these elements help to produce a more therapeutic individualized treatment plan, what activities could you engage in to integrate them into your "automatic" thinking patterns?

2. Write a nursing diagnosis, prognosis and set of treatment directives. Show them to a nursing colleague and ask the person to think out loud, interpret what you have written, and plan how to implement them. Ask the person to raise any questions as to the behavior that is expected, what the directives mean, and how to go about implementing them. Listen without interrupting, interpreting, or giving any cues by your facial expression or body language during the time your colleague is reacting to the plan. Allow your written words to speak for themselves. Then, together, edit the plan so that it is mutually understood.

3. Notice how other nurses communicate their treatment directives to you orally and in writing. Could you carry them out exactly as they were communicated? Critique them in terms of their clarity and specificity. What did you learn from this experience? How will it modify the way in which you communicate your treatment directives?

4. Experiment repeatedly with deliberately contrasting general nursing directives and precise, specific directives until you become very aware of the important place that precision in language plays in communicating the treatment plan.

References

AXELSSON K: *Eating Problems and Nutritional Status after Stroke.* Advanced Nursing and Medicine, University of Umea, Sweden: Umea University Medical Dissertations. New Series No 218-ISSN 0346–6612, 1988.

BROWN M, CARRIERI V, JANSON-BJERKLIE S, DODD M: Lung cancer and dyspnea: the patient's perspective. *Oncology Nursing Forum* 13:25, 1986.

BULECHECK G, McCLOSKEY J (eds): *Nursing Interventions: Treatments for Nursing Diagnoses.* Philadelphia: W.B. Saunders, 1985.

CARNEVALI D: *Sykepleieplanlegging.* Oslo: Gyldendal Norsk Forlag, 1992.

CARNEVALI D, REINER A: *The Cancer Experience: Nursing Diagnosis and Management.* Philadelphia: J.B. Lippincott, 1990.

CARNEVALI D: Daily living and functional health status: A perspective for nursing diagnosis and treatment. *Archives of Psychiatric Nursing* 2(6):333, 1988.

CARNEVALI D: Health care for the elderly: Nursing's area of accountability. In Carnevali D, Patrick M (eds): *Nursing Management for the Elderly*. 3rd ed. Philadelphia: J.B. Lippincott, 1993.

CARPENITO L: *Nursing Diagnosis: Application to Clinical Practice*, 4th ed. Philadelphia: J.B. Lippincott, 1991.

CHRISMAN NJ: Culture-sensitive nursing care. In Patrick M, Woods S, Craven R, Rokosky J, Bruno P (eds): *Medical-Surgical Nursing: Pathophysiological Concepts*. 2nd ed. Philadelphia: J.B. Lippincott, 1991, pp. 34–47.

CORCORAN S: Decision analysis: a step-by-step guide for making clinical decisions. *Nursing and Health Care* 7:149–154, 1986. (a)

CORCORAN S: Task complexity and nursing expertise as factors in decision making. *Nursing Research* 35:107–112, 1986. (b)

CORCORAN S: Expert and novice nurses' use of knowledge to plan for pain control: How clinicians make their decisions. *The American Journal of Hospice Care* 3(6):37–41, 1986. (c)

CRANDALL L: Daily living with Alzheimer's disease and daily living with behavioral problems. In Carnevali D, Patrick M (eds): *Nursing Management for the Elderly*. 3rd ed. Philadelphia: J.B. Lippincott, 1993.

GOLD W: Dyspnea. In Blacklow R (ed): *MacBryde's Signs and Symptoms*. 6th ed. Philadelphia: J.B. Lippincott, 1983.

HAYES-ROTH B, HAYES-ROTH F: A cognitive model of planning. *Cognitive Science* 3:275–310, 1979.

HEIMLICH HJ: Rehabilitation of swallowing after stroke. *Annals of Otology, Rhinology and Laryngology* 92:357–359, 1983.

HOFFART N: Renal failure. In Carnevali D, Patrick M (eds): *Nursing Management for the Elderly*. 3rd ed. Philadelphia: J.B. Lippincott, 1993.

KLEINMUTZ B: The processing of information by man and machine. In Kleinmutz B (ed): *The Formal Representation of Human Judgment*. New York: Wiley, 1968.

LAREAU S: Respiratory problems. In Carnevali D, Patrick M (eds): *Nursing Management for the Elderly*. 3rd ed. Philadelphia: J.B. Lippincott, 1993.

LEE K: Nursing care of patients with disturbances in arousal and sleep patterns. In Patrick M, Woods S, Craven R, Rokosky J, Bruno P (eds): *Medical-Surgical Nursing: Pathophysiological Concepts*. 2nd ed. Philadelphia: J.B. Lippincott, 1991.

MCGUIRE C: Medical problem-solving: A critique of the literature. *Journal of Medical Education* 60:587–595, 1985.

MCGUIRE C, BABBOTT D: Simulation technique in the measurement of problem-solving skills. *Journal of Educational Measurement* 4:1–10, 1967.

NARAYAN S: *Heuristic Reasoning About Uncertainty in a Clinical Nursing Task*. University of Minnesota: Doctoral Dissertation, 1990.

OZUNA JH: Nursing strategies for common neurological problems: Nursing diagnosis, interventions, evaluation. In Patrick M, Woods S, Craven R, Rokosky J, Bruno P (eds): *Medical-Surgical Nursing: Pathophysiological Concepts*. 2nd ed. Philadelphia: J.B. Lippincott, 1991, pp. 1155–1175.

PAYNE J: Contingent decision behavior. *Psychological Bulletin* 92:382–402, 1982.

PEPLAU H: A working definition of anxiety. In Burd S, Marshall M (eds): *Some Clinical Approaches to Psychiatric Nursing*. New York: Macmillan, 1963.

RAIFFA H. *Decision Analysis: Introductory Lectures on Choice under Uncertainty.* Reading, MA: Addison-Wesley, 1968.

THOMAS M, SANGER E: Diagnostic clusters, holism and reductionism. Paper presented at Theory and Research-based Psychosocial Nursing Practice Conference. Seattle, WA: Department of Psychosocial Nursing, University of Washington, July 12–14, 1989.

TVERSKY A, KAHNEMAN D: The framing of decisions and psychology of choice. *Science* 211:453–458, 1981.

WHITLEY G: Anxiety (mild, moderate, severe, extreme/panic). In McFarland G, Thomas M: *Psychiatric Mental Health Nursing Application of the Nursing Process.* Philadelphia: J.B. Lippincott, 1991.

6

Factors Affecting Clinical Judgment and Decision Making

It is easy to think of diagnosing as a rather cut-and-dried objective process of taking in data, classifying them, and assigning a label to what is observed. In reality, there are many factors influencing the process. Some of these factors are internal to the clinician while some are external. Many of these factors cannot be controlled by the clinician. Still, it is wise to be aware of them since they can actually shape the judgments and decisions made and thus ultimately affect the care that patients and their families receive.

Discipline-specific Factors Affecting Diagnosing

One obvious influence on diagnosing and deciding on treatment is the focus of training and experience the novice clinician receives in order to become an expert in a particular health care field. Basic education and training will determine the clinician's subsequent perspective, knowledge base, language, diagnostic taxonomic categories, role expectations, and relationships.

Discipline-specific Perspective for Diagnosis and Treatment

A central goal of the curriculum and clinical experience in preparing a member of a given health profession is the development of expertise in diagnosing and treating patient situations from the perspective of that specific discipline. For example, basic professional training prepares

- physicians to prevent, diagnose, and treat pathophysiology;
- nutritionists to deal with nutrients, food selection and preparation, and eating to promote health or optimum nutrition in the face of pathology or treatment side effects;
- pharmacists to assist people in effective use of prescribed or over-the-counter medications;
- dentists to promote oral health and to diagnose and to treat teeth and supporting/ surrounding structures that are damaged by pathology or side effects of medical treatments;
- nurses for a dual focus in their clinical practice: 1) adequate knowledge of pathology, pathophysiology, psychopathology, and medical treatment to safely carry out delegated medical care, 2) expert knowledge on human responses to health states and related experiences, dimensions of daily living that affect and are affected by the health situation, and the associated external resources.

Beyond basic training, clinical specialty training can further narrow and deepen a clinician's perspective for diagnosis and treatment. Many nurses move from being generalists to becoming specialists in oncology, psychiatry, cardiology, obstetrics, endocrinology, etc., or even some subspecialty within a clinical specialty. They are then prepared to diagnose and treat both common and uncommon problems within their specialty but may at the same time decrease their attention and assignment of significance to data that reflect problems outside that field. For example:

A 28-year-old woman with schizophrenia is in her third trimester of pregnancy and approaching her due date. On this particular morning she talks of a devil and becomes increasingly agitated. She does not indicate any discomfort or pain through facial grimacing or verbal expression but periodically stops pacing and rocks back and forth. The initial focus of the psychiatric nurse might be on the alteration in thought processes and the bizarre behavior associated with schizophrenia. An obstetric nurse, on the other hand, might interpret the rocking and agitation as being associated with beginning labor.

The potential for narrowed vision or for ineffectiveness in diagnosing in an unfamiliar field is recognized when psychiatric clinical specialists serve as consultants to nurses on general medical or surgical units, critical care units and obstetric units. Conversely, assistance of nurses on these other units may be sought by psychiatric nurses. Even within a specialized field, nurses may develop a particular subspecialization or interest. For example:

A man is receiving cisplatin as treatment for his lung cancer. He is a highly anxious person, very frightened. He is accompanied by an equally tense wife.

An oncology nurse who has specialized in chemotherapy may focus on safe administration of drugs and management of the patient's responses during the time of administration (Goodman, 1991, pp. 291–320).

A nurse who has done advanced work in nausea and vomiting associated with chemotherapy might focus on factors that predict difficulties with this side effect of treatment (Rhodes, Watson and Johnson, 1986) and strategies for minimizing them as well as management of daily living for patient and family to most effectively deal with these uncomfortable, persistent side effects (Carnevali and Reiner, 1990, pp. 142–160).

A nurse who has specialized in human responses to uncertainty might tend to look more at these aspects of the patient and family situation (Mishel, 1988).

A home care nurse might focus on the wife's needs as primary caregiver and food preparer (Carnevali and Reiner, 1990, pp. 150, 157–159).

Some diagnosticians may become "narrow" in their valuing of other diagnostic perspectives, believing that their own perspective is the only one that really matters and failing to value others' diagnostic perspectives and activities. It becomes important for a clinician in any health care field to consider the education and training of diagnosticians in other fields—to recognize the contribution each one is prepared to make in a given patient situation. It is also wise to realize the limitations in diagnostic perspective and expertise each clinician experiences as a result of discipline-specific training—one's own and that of others. For example:

A nurse was attending a workshop on nursing diagnosis. As part of the learning experiences, participants worked with a case in which a previously healthy, vigorous, independent woman in her early eighties had suffered a fractured hip that was treated by pinning. Her postoperative course was normal and prognosis for healing and returning function was good. The nursing diagnosis dealt with her distressing concern that she would be sent to a nursing home and would not be able to return to her own home and her independent lifestyle.

That evening the nurse shared the case data with her husband who was an orthopedist. He provided a medical diagnosis giving his opinion that the woman had nothing to worry about, her prognosis seemed very good for her age. When shown the diagnosis the nurses had developed, he indicated that it was no diagnosis at all because it addressed the situation and not the pathology.

Both basic and advanced discipline-specific education shape the diagnostic point of view and expertise that is given priority and valued. For the patient's sake it is important to be aware of both the advantages and limitations of discipline-specific diagnostic orientation and expertise.

Influence of the Discipline's Knowledge Base on Diagnosing

There is no question that what a diagnostician "knows" affects what the person is prepared to attend to and diagnose the diagnostic approach. For example:

A nurse who does not recognize and know that circadian rhythms result in reduced ability of patients with coronary artery disease to tolerate exercise within four hours of wakening and also result in higher risk of cardiac arrest in this same time period may permit activities or stressful visitors during this time of increased vulnerability (Muller et al., 1987; Lemmer, 1989; Joy, Pollard and Nunan, 1982);

A nurse who does not recognize the body language of a premature infant will have difficulty in diagnosing the stressors or needs the infant is expressing and thus be ineffective in establishing effective patterns in daily living;

A nurse who does not identify signs of role ambiguity or role conflict can fail to diagnose and treat a response to a health state or situation that may be very responsive to nursing treatment.

Knowledge, theoretical and clinical, affect both diagnosis and treatment planning. Nursing knowledge in the United States tends to be organized in terms of categories of human responses to health states or situations (see Table 6-1). Thus, nurses are being trained to recognize, understand and treat health situations using a body of knowledge with this focus and structure. Knowledge from other fields (e.g., anthropology, biochemistry, biological structure, ecology, economics, ethics, ethnicity, genetics, gerontology, growth and development, law, medicine, microbiology, nutrition, pathology, pharmacology, physiology, political science, psychology, psychiatry, sociology, technology) is fitted into the nursing perspective and structure.

The language used to describe clinical phenomena grows out of the knowledge base and the way it is structured. Thus, different disciplines may use different words to describe the same phenomenon. For example:

A patient is complaining of severe substernal pain that wakens him nightly. The NANDA category would be altered comfort—pain or sleep pattern disturbance; the medical label would be resting angina.

A patient with a history of diabetes mellitus is complaining of chronic severe burning sensation in the hands and feet. The nursing category would be altered comfort—pain; the medical label would be diabetic peripheral neuropathy—specifically, glove and stocking paresthesia.

On the other hand, the knowledge base may permit one discipline to diagnose phenomena that tend not to be addressed by another. For example:

A blind man in his mid-thirties who lives in a residence for individuals with low incomes is to be admitted to the hospital for some diagnostic tests. His constant companion is his seeing-eye dog. He is becoming highly anxious about the care of his dog during his absence, but as a very independent and somewhat isolated person, is unable to ask others to help him. The nurse who oversees health care of residents in the building, diagnoses the problem and negotiates with the man and another occupant of the residence who is willing to be taught how to work with and care for a "working dog" during the patient's absence. The physician who was seeking to diagnose pathophysiological problems did not think about the difficulty of appropriately maintaining and caring for a seeing eye dog.

A nurse in the coronary care unit diagnoses secondary insomnia associated with care procedures and has knowledge about the role of sleep in the healing process (Lee, 1991). She arranges to group procedures and restrict disruptions when the patient is in a normal sleep cycle. Physicians and medical students more concerned with the cardiac pathology and their own schedules have not paid attention to sleep problems.

The discipline's language may also determine the level of precision that is the standard or is usual in describing etiology, manifestations, or diagnoses. These levels of precision occur in qualitative, quantitative, and labeling areas. Discipline-specific orientation to precision may be reflected in the thinking and language norms for members of that health care group. Probably biomedical areas foster the

TABLE 6-1 Comparison of Classification Systems for Nursing and Medical and Social Work Diagnoses.

Nursing[a]	Medicine[b]	Social Work[c]
Exchanging	Infectious and parasitic diseases	*Problems in social role functioning*
Communicating	Neoplasms	Control/power
Relating	Endocrine, nutritional metabolic, and immune diseases	Conflict/ambivalence
Valuing	Mental diseases	Responsibility/performance expectation
Choosing	Diseases of the nervous and sense organs	Dependence/reactive
Moving	Diseases of the circulatory system	Independence/proactive
Perceiving	Diseases of the respiratory system	Status/status change
Knowing	Diseases of the digestive system	Separation/loss
Feeling	Diseases of the genitourinary system	Isolation/withdrawal
	Pregnancy, childbirth, and puerperia	Intimidation/victimization
	Diseases of the skin and subcutaneous tissue	Mixed
	Diseases of the musculoskeletal system and connective tissue	Other (specify)
	Congenital abnormalities	*Environmental systems and problem areas*
	Certain conditions originating in perinatal period	Economic/basic needs system
	Symptoms, signs, and ill-defined conditions	Education/training system
	Injury and poisoning	Judicial/legal system
		Health, safety, and social service system
	Supplementary clarification	Voluntary association system
	Class of factors influencing health status and contact with health services	Affectional support system
	Class of external causes of injury and poisoning	

[a]From Kim MJ, McFarland G, McLane A (eds). *Classification of Nursing Diagnoses: Proceedings of the Fifth National Conference.* St Louis, MO: Mosby, 1984, p 29; Fitzpatrick J: Taxonomy II: Definitions and development, *Classification of Nursing Diagnoses: Proceedings of the Ninth Conference.* Philadelphia: J.B. Lippincott, 1991, pp 23–29.

[b]From *The International Classification of Diseases*, 9th revision. Clinical Revision. 2nd ed. Washington, DC: US Dept of Health and Human Services, 1980.

[c]From Williams J, Karls J, Wandrei K: The Person-in-Environment (PIE) system for describing problems of social functioning. *Hospital and Community Psychiatry* 40(11):1125–1127, 1989, p 1126.

greatest expectation of precision, as illustrated by laboratory values measured in nanograms, and electrocardiogram tracings measured in millimeters.

In the nursing literature some diagnostic concepts have been developed that permit certain levels of precision in descriptors. For example:

Anxiety: Peplau described four different levels of anxiety, their manifestations and implications for nursing treatment (1963). Subsequent nursing research has documented these levels of anxiety, their effects and rationale for treatment in a variety of health states (Whitley, 1991).

Pain: Using work done in other fields, nursing researchers have tested descriptors of the nature, distribution, occurrence patterns and level of pain (both acute and chronic) and have incorporated these into their diagnosis of problems managing daily living in the presence of precisely described pain (Feldman, 1991; Carnevali and Reiner, 1990). One oncology unit used a 10-point analogue scale and philosophy of pain control. They believed that patients on their unit were not to routinely manage the challenges of daily living with prolonged pain in excess of a self-rated 3.

Suffering: In addition to the concept of pain, the concept of suffering has also been developed as a separate area for differential diagnosis (Benedict, 1989; Duclow, 1988). This is an area for diagnosis that can be applied to patients or those who share the health experience. Unlike pain, there is no research on quantitative levels of distress associated with the concept of suffering.

Taxonomic Categories

The taxonomic structure for labeling health problems of individuals and groups unquestionably affects diagnosing behavior. It offers or tends to close off options for diagnosing. For example, some nurses believe that they cannot diagnose any problem not yet specifically accepted for testing in the NANDA taxonomy.

Initial taxonomic systems in health care were disease oriented, as illustrated by the title of the reference most widely used, *International Classification of Diseases* (*ICD*), currently moving toward a 10th edition. Table 6-1 illustrates different perspectives for diagnosing by comparing three systems: Taxonomy I, Revised of the North American Nursing Diagnosis Association (NANDA); the International Classification of Disease, Ninth Revision; and the Person-in-Environment system from the field of social work. Time, clinical research, and experience have permitted medical taxonomists to develop increasingly precise diagnostic categories and diagnoses, as illustrated by the 1,186 pages of diagnostic categories in *ICD,* Volume I. NANDA, with only a 20-year history, has had less time to develop nursing's taxonomic structure. Many phenomena have yet to be researched and incorporated into the NANDA taxonomy and highly specific taxonomic levels remain to be developed. For a full listing of Taxonomy I Revised (1990) taxonomic categories, see Appendix A. For a listing of Human Responses of Concern for Psychiatric Mental Health Nursing Practice, see Appendix B.

At present, if nurses feel compelled to limit themselves to taxonomic categories currently "accepted for clinical testing," some problems can remain undiagnosed or diagnosed at a level too imprecise to provide for individualized treatment.

See *Exercise Set 1* for activities exploring the effect of disciplines on diagnostic perspective.

Effect of Role Expectations on Nurses' Diagnostic and Treatment Planning Behavior

Role expectations in the work setting influence workers' behavior. In the area of nursing diagnosis and treatment planning, role expectations emerge both from inside and outside the nursing profession. These expectations influence the priorities and values that workers place on diagnostic and treatment planning behaviors as well as the way they carry out associated activities.

Nursing's Self-expectations Regarding Diagnosis and Treatment Planning

The nursing profession itself has developed expectations for nurses' behavior and activities in the area of nursing diagnosis and treatment planning. These are expressed in both formal and informal ways.

Formal Role Expectations

In the United States, accreditation of institutions and agencies requires nurses to provide evidence of planned nursing care. State nurse licensure acts include requirements of skill in and implementation of nursing diagnosis and treatment planning. Failure to engage in appropriate and effective nursing diagnosis and treatment planning can result in disciplinary action. The American Nurses Association has designated the North American Nursing Diagnosis Association (NANDA) as the official body to develop nursing's diagnostic taxonomy. Curricula and textbooks are organized to foster diagnostic and treatment planning knowledge and skills. Many now use taxonomic headings as an organizing structure.

In clinical settings many nursing departments have a standard that nursing assessments, diagnoses, and plans are to be documented within 8–24 hours of admission or of the first home visit. Nursing home residents are expected to have care plans that are updated at specified intervals. Quality assurance groups audit records to evaluate documented performance.

See *Exercise 2-1* for activities exploring formal role expectations and their communication.

Informal Role Expectations

In actual day-to-day practice, there is more variability in role expectations regarding the priority and significance assigned to nursing diagnosis and treatment planning. Role expectations can range from a low priority among activities and skills to being a valued and central part of the nursing role.

A low priority and value for diagnostic behavior is sometimes evidenced. For example:

> Nurses give positive feedback to their colleagues for their expertise in making clinical judgments in the medical domain but make jokes about the accreditation requirements for documenting nursing diagnoses and treatment plans. Diagnoses and treatments are documented more to please administration, and less to benefit patients, by identifying, addressing, and communicating individual patient problems.

> Nurses routinely assign the same standard general nursing diagnoses and plans of care to all patients and families who have a common pathology, even though the responses to their health state and situation may vary widely.

In other nursing settings, both informal and formal role expectations are that nurses will exhibit a high degree of accountability and expertise in nursing diagnosis. On these units one might see that:

> The contribution that nursing diagnoses and treatments are making to patient and family well-being is regularly acknowledged. Patients and families are involved in all aspects of the process whenever this is feasible and appropriate.

> Nursing case conferences are held to address situations that are difficult to diagnose and treat; participants are prepared to be challenged and to defend their judgments and decisions.

> Nursing excellence is evaluated in self and others on the basis of diagnostic and treatment planning expertise; mentoring and support is offered to nurses with less experience and expertise.

> Nursing diagnoses and treatments are as integral to change-of-shift reports and assignment conferences as medical diagnoses and treatment.

Both formal and informal role expectations of other nurses about diagnostic and treatment planning behavior in the work setting can strongly influence an individual nurse's diagnostic behavior.

See *Exercise 2-2 through 2-4* for activities exploring the work setting's informal role expectations and their communication as well as one's own expectations.

Role Expectations of Other Groups

In addition to the influence of professional self-expectations, nurses' diagnostic behavior can also be affected by others involved in patient health care situations.

Physicians

Physicians can either value or not value nursing diagnoses and treatments. Traditionally, physicians have viewed nurses as a means of implementing delegated medical functions (Prescott and Bowen, 1985; Prescott, Dennis, and Jacox, 1987; Stein, Watts and Howell, 1990). Now, nursing roles incorporate dual clinical responsibilities in which nurses: 1) continue their traditional role of implementing delegated medical functions, and 2) diagnose and prescribe within the nursing domain. Many physicians currently recognize and value the distinct contribution that nursing perspective brings to health care and the way in which it frees them to practice medicine (Stein, Watts, and Howell, 1990). However, other physicians are confused and angry with nurses' expectations of autonomy when they practice within nursing's self-defined nursing domain (Stein, Watts, and Howell, 1990).

Nurses can experience both positive and negative reactions as they diagnose and treat within the nursing domain. There can be positive physician feedback in the form of consistent support in general and in individual patient situations. On the other hand, nurses can find that physicians ignore or even negate or ridicule documented plans and diagnostic behavior. Much depends on the level of confidence and trust physicians have for the competence of the specific nurse in delegated medical functions as well as in the nursing domain (Prescott and Bowen, 1985). It also may depend on the manner in which the nurse presents ideas (Prescott and Bowen, 1985; Stein, 1967).

See *Exercise 3-1* for activities to identify physicians, responses to nursing diagnostic and treatment planning activities.

Other Health Care Groups

Health care workers in other fields, such as occupational therapy, social work, nutrition, and physical therapy, may also either value or not value nurses' diagnostic and treatment efforts. At times, professional control and "turf" can become an issue where there is overlap of interests. On the other hand, diagnoses and treatment can often be improved by the incorporation of data, knowledge, or judgments from an allied field and by integration of diagnoses and treatment plans.

See *Exercise Set 3* for activities to identify the responses of other health care provider groups to nursing diagnostic and treatment planning activities.

Patients and Families

Feedback from patients and families can influence nursing diagnostic and treatment planning behavior. By their very nature, nursing diagnoses and treatment involve patients and families in a participatory relationship, so their attitudes toward these nursing activities become important. When patients and families are aware of the diagnoses and treatment plans and find them accurate and helpful, support for these nursing activities tends to be positive and strong. Even patients or families whose initial insight or status does not permit them to agree with or accept the nursing diagnoses may in hindsight appreciate the expertise in nursing care the plans represent. When nurses experience this kind of feedback, there is increased enthusiasm for the activities.

Lawyers

One other profession can directly affect nursing diagnostic and treatment planning behavior—the legal profession. Lawsuits involving health care often address nursing care and documentation. In order to prevent legal difficulties, lawyers may be called in as consultants on nursing documentation. Their guidelines and recommendations may determine nurses' sense of freedom, and accountability in diagnosing and, at times the language that can or cannot be safely used.

Government, Third Party Payers, and Accrediting Agencies

Regulations that guide nursing diagnosis, treatment planning and evaluation of response arise from several sources, including federal, state and local governmental agencies, health insurance companies and accrediting agencies. These regulations tend to guide what diagnostic and treatment activities are to be undertaken and when they are to be done. Nursing diagnostic and treatment behavior is evaluated through audits of documentation, interviews with patients, and inspections by accrediting bodies. Individuals who inspect or audit a nursing department and interpret regulations can vary widely in their own expertise and experience, in diagnosis and treatment planning in clinical settings. On the other hand, nurses in institutions or agencies who are skilled and confident in their nursing diagnoses and treatment plans often are able to provide data and rationale to support their care and documentation even though it may vary from the regulations. Nurses who lack skill or feel threatened may seek security in bureaucratic expectations even when there is a conflict between these and what the individual patient and family may truly need.

Because governmental agencies are sources of funding for health care institutions, they create a powerful influence on nursing behavior. There can be strong administrative pressure to meet the letter of the guidelines.

See **Exercises 3-3 and 3-4** for activities to identify the influences of legal and accreditation bodies on diagnostic and treatment planning activities.

Influence of Clientele on Diagnostic Behavior

The nature of the clientele and their health status and situations exert major influences on data collection, diagnosis, and treatment planning. This is particularly true when a nurse has been caring for patients and families who have common health problems or situations, nursing care is centered around a specific type of treatment, or duration of health care is the common thread.

Effect on Diagnosing of Clientele Having Similar Health Problems

Nurses who regularly care for patients and families who share a particular diagnosis or complex of diagnoses tend to focus on and become expert in identifying nursing problems associated with this health situation. Some will be problems that occur commonly; others will be rare but of such consequence that nurses remain alert for them.

Day-by-day encounters over time with patients and families who experience similar health problems create for nurses a strong library of theoretical/clinical knowledge and patient instances in long term memory. The range of situations and responses creates a pool of experience that enables the nurse to identify commonalities but also to recognize variations and contrasts. For example:

> Neonatal nurses are seeking to learn to differentiate between the kinds of manifestations shown by babies who are fussy because they are experiencing withdrawal from crack cocaine from those who are fussy from other causes (Tanner, Benner, Chesla, and Gordon, submitted for publication).

While knowledge from semantic memory forms a theoretical background, clinical knowledge and finesse in observation undoubtedly draw on the pool of patient instance scripts stored over time.

As nurses develop patterns of assessment, diagnosis, and treatment in their specialty that efficiently address the needs and problems of a particular clientele, they can become less attentive to or expert in diagnosing and treating human responses and situations that fall outside of this clinical specialty. For example:

> Contrast the problems associated with response to health situations involving

- Alzheimer's disease
- autism,
- cancer—initial stages, advanced-metastatic,
- cystic fibrosis,
- stroke,
- insulin dependent diabetes,
- pregnancy,
- prematurity,
- schizophrenia,
- sexually transmitted diseases,
- urinary incontinence.

It can be seen that a nurse who has worked with premature infants for years might feel ill-prepared to address the problems of patients and families facing the challenges of Alzheimer's disease or diabetes. Sometimes, there is further specialization in terms of caring for individuals of a particular age group who have these health problems, such as the child with cancer and the adult with cancer, or the child with autism and the adult with schizophrenia.

Nurses often become specialized in working with patients and families who must live with particular health states and their treatment. Their ongoing exposure to the challenges involved in living with these conditions tends to cause a certain mind-set for diagnoses and treatment modalities they are prepared to consider.

See *Exercise Set 4* for activities to identify the effect of nurses' clientele on their diagnostic and treatment planning activities.

Effect on Diagnosing of Working with a Specialized Medical Therapy

Some nurses specialize in working with patients and families while they are dealing with the challenges of particular forms of medical therapy, for example,

- chemotherapy,
- radiation,
- surgery,
- rehabilitation,
- aversion therapy,
- behavior modification,
- organ transplantation.

Here the diagnostic perspective moves to the capacities of patients and families to respond to challenges in daily living posed by the therapy more than the pathology. It is often a nursing specialty within a clinical specialty that can bring with it a narrowing of focus.

Influence of Duration of Nursing Contact on Diagnostic Behavior

The duration of anticipated contact for offering nursing care also influences diagnostic behavior. When nurses have only a brief, one-time contact with a patient and family or when the known duration of contact will be short, the breadth of assessment, diagnosis and treatment will be narrower than when nursing care will continue to be given over longer periods of time. Contrast the breadth of nursing diagnostic focus in the following situations:

- A healthy adult having a hernia repaired in a day surgery setting.
- A 7-year-old child just diagnosed as having diabetes mellitus.
- A 35-year-old, healthy male entering the emergency room for removal of a foreign object from his eye.
- A 55-year-old woman and her husband admitted to a renal dialysis program for training in home dialysis.

- A 60-year-old woman with diagnosed Parkinson's disease living with her 65-year-old husband who has coronary artery disease.
- A 28-year-old man diagnosed as having AIDS.

Nurses vary their data collection, diagnosis and treatment to adjust to the nursing care that is needed or feasible and the opportunities available to provide the care.

Effect on Diagnosing of "Knowing" the Person[1]

Another factor affecting judgments made about the patient and the situation is that of genuinely "knowing" the person and the family—learning what each one is experiencing, what it means to them, and how they are responding (Tanner, Benner, Chesla, and Gordon, submitted for publication). Knowing a patient can involve recognition and understanding of the individual's subtle, specific physiological patterns of responses to the situation, to medical treatment, or nursing activities. It also involves knowing the patient and family members as individuals and understanding how the health situation is truly affecting them, their interaction, and their lives from their point of view.

Knowing a patient and family in this way arises from a nurse's belief that nursing integrates personal concern for patients and their families with professional caring for them. Then, beyond any formal nursing assessment, ongoing interaction will be characterized by this concerned, expert attention to the patient and others closely involved in the health situation.

It can be seen that nurses' beliefs and values, associated with observation and clinical judgments, will be influential factors in their approach to both initial and ongoing assessments. Some nurses value "going by the book," meeting the requirements of data collection indicated on the nursing assessment form. Some nurses may value most a focus on pathophysiology and response to medical activities. Some nurses will value using each patient and family encounter to build trust and come to know and understand those involved as a basis for protecting them, advocating for them, and providing the most effective, personalized and caring nursing treatment possible.

Influence of Setting and Equipment on Diagnostic Behavior

There are a variety of physical factors in the clinical setting that strongly influence the focus and nature of nurses' diagnostic behavior. These include the physical

[1]Material in this section was derived from personal communication from Christine Tanner, Professor, Department of Adult Health and Illness Nursing, Oregon Health Sciences University. It is based on a research project undertaken by C. Tanner, P. Benner, C. Chesla, and D. Gordon.

setting itself, equipment available for collecting data, computers, forms, and clinical assignments.

Physical Setting

The setting in which assessment and diagnosis take place can affect diagnostic behavior. Contrast the effect of surroundings for assessment-diagnosis in each of the following situations:

- A nurse-midwife preparing to help a woman and her family engage in the birthing experience in the home and the same clinical situation in a hospital labor and delivery room.
- A busy emergency clinic.
- An admission desk for an ambulatory care surgery unit.
- A two-bed room on an oncology unit.
- An apartment in a retirement home.
- A county jail unit.

The physical setting, the people in it, and the surrounding pace of activities can all affect assessment-diagnostic behavior.

Equipment

The normally available equipment is another source of influence. In some settings very little diagnostic equipment is available; in others state-of-the-art equipment is available and nurses are expected to use it. For example:

In some settings nurses are involved in answering patient's phone calls. The only form of data they have available on which to make clinical judgments is auditory data. Their skill in diagnosing and making treatment decisions is based on their ability to: 1) enable the caller to provide accurate, precise descriptions of what is happening and what they are experiencing, and 2) interpret tone of voice, rate of speech, speech patterns, breathing patterns, and nonspeech sounds.

In a coronary care unit the nurse has access to all the auditory cues plus the opportunity to see and touch the patient, listen to heart and breath sounds, obtain blood pressure readings, read the monitor data, and obtain data on blood gases and enzymes and other laboratory findings.

This is not to say that the nurse whose only contact is through a telephone will make a less accurate diagnosis, only that the equipment, and therefore the data available, are different.

When monitors and machines become the source of data, sometimes the focus of the diagnostician's attention shifts to equipment and away from those generating the data and what they are experiencing. It is as if patterns and numbers produced are more solid, real, and believable than the person. This can affect diagnostic behavior.

Computers

Computers can be useful in diagnosis and treatment, or they can create real limitations. In some work settings nurses are limited to the data, nursing diagnoses, and treatments that have been programmed into the institution's nursing computer system. The quality of these programs varies, and as a result, so will the diagnoses. If nurses become comfortable with this requirement, they may cease to attend to findings, diagnoses, and treatment options not included in the computer program.

See *Exercise Set 5* for activities exploring the influence of equipment on nursing diagnostic and treatment decisions.

Forms

Data collection forms and other documentation forms also influence the diagnostic process for nurses. They dictate the focus of assessment—possibly the areas and sequence of data to be collected as well as the space to be devoted to any particular category of data. Some clinical settings use checklists of diagnoses and data that can be documented. Others have categories and blanks that must be filled in—the expectation being that these data will be collected whether they are relevant or not. Some have descriptors that must be used. Still others are quite free-form, depending on the expertise of the nurse. In each case, the form influences the diagnostic practice of the nurse in some way.

See *Exercise Set 6* for activities to explore the influence of forms on diagnostic and treatment decisions.

Assignments

Case assignments affect diagnostic behavior. Nurses on high-turnover surgical units who regularly have multiple admissions will have less time to engage in assessment-diagnosis than those who work on an oncology unit with lower turnover and where patients tend to stay longer and be readmitted. Oncology nurses expect to come to know their patients and families well and will seek data to serve as a baseline for readmissions and for assisting patients with their responses during the intervals at home between admissions.

Care assignments, in which nurses are held accountable for diagnosis and treatment of a case load of patients over time, tend to generate a sense of accountability for the totality of patient care. This in turn can affect the priority and effort a nurse brings to diagnosing and planning care for a caseload. Assignments which fluctuate unpredictably from one case load to another tend to lead to a view of diagnosis and treatment planning as isolated tasks that are required behavior—it becomes difficult to see the results of one's diagnostic and treatment planning efforts.

See *Exercise Set 7* for activities to explore the effect of nurse assignments on diagnostic and treatment planning activities.

Summary

Often nurses have little control over environmental factors that can affect diagnostic and treatment planning behavior. Still, it is wise to be aware of their potential influence and occasionally to stand back and determine:

- how one's behavior is being affected;
- whether this effect is resulting in more or less effective diagnosing and treatment planning;
- what accommodations or compensatory adjustments could be made to diagnose and treat effectively within the setting;
- what changes in the environment could be made to permit or foster more effective diagnosing and treatment planning.

Characteristics of the Individual Diagnostician

In addition to the external factors that shape the diagnostician's behavior and skill, there are intrapersonal factors as well. Some of these are long term, ongoing capabilities or attributes. Others are transient, affecting diagnostic and treatment planning behavior only at a particular point in time.

Long Term Characteristics of the Diagnostician

Personal attributes and capabilities that vary among nurses have the potential to influence diagnostic and treatment planning abilities. These activities involve noticing data in the clinical situation, assigning meaning (words, impressions, or numbers) to the incoming data, considering possible diagnostic explanations for what has been noticed, collecting more data, and eventually assigning the findings a diagnosis. This suggests the need for:

- ability to notice or sense both obvious and subtle, disguised cues in the situation;
- a command of knowledge and language that results in precise descriptors for or impressions of incoming data;
- capacity to judge which cues are important and which should be given lower priority or ignored;
- organization of knowledge in long term memory that permits retrieval of relevant diagnostic concepts;
- recognition and valuing of patient instances for their variability as well as commonalities;
- ability to synthesize findings and knowledge as a basis for making clinical judgments about diagnosis and treatment;

- capacity to tolerate ambiguity or delay when there are insufficient data to permit an immediate diagnosis;
- willingness to persist in observation and thinking until the observed phenomena can be diagnosed or ruled out (decision that the problem does not exist);
- expectations and acceptance of the dynamic, changing quality of patient responses and situations in the nursing domain resulting in the need to maintain watchfulness and modify diagnoses, prognoses, and treatments;
- assigning value to coming to "know" the person and what is being experienced in a sensitive and concerned way.

Nurses can vary initially in their basic capabilities in these areas. Patterns of growth in each of these areas as a result of greater knowledge and additional experience can also vary. Thus, individual nurses vary in their capacities and abilities for diagnosis and treatment planning.

Additionally, clinical experience can make a nurse highly expert in diagnosis and treatment planning in one clinical area and less expert in others. Diagnostic prowess is a profile, not a steady state.

Temporary Intrapersonal Factors

In addition to the more enduring characteristics and abilities of the diagnostician, there are also temporary conditions that can affect capacity to make clinical judgments. These include:

- status of one's sense organs, e.g., misplacing one's contact lenses;
- being physically fatigued, e.g., assessing a newly admitted patient at the end of a hectic 12-hour shift on the last evening before days off;
- feeling ill or in pain, e.g., experiencing severe menstrual cramps;
- being emotionally distraught, e.g., highly anxious, angry, or depressed.

Any one or more of these personal states can interfere with one's capacity to attend to data and engage in the critical thinking that is central to diagnosing and treating patients.

See *Exercise Set 8* for activity to explore one's own characteristics as they affect diagnostic and treatment capabilities.

Complexity of the Diagnostic Task

Another factor influencing diagnostic activities is the complexity of the diagnostic task. Diagnosing involves making a clinical judgment about the unobservable nature of clients and their situations based on data presented (Tanner, 1984). The probabilistic relationship between available cues and the client's situation makes diagnosing an uncertain and complicated activity (Fox, 1980).

Nursing's diagnostic activities require ascertaining the presence or absence of an abnormal state or difficulty based on one or more cues and differentiation between two or more abnormal states or types of difficulties (Hammond, 1966).

Influence of the Nature of Cues and Their Availability

Complexity in the diagnostic task is associated with accessibility of cues and other cue characteristics. These include:

Number of cues: In general, the greater the number of cues present in the situation, the greater the complexity of the diagnostic task.

Reliability of cues: Some cues are strongly linked to particular client situations; others have a weak association.

Redundancy of cues: Repetitive cues, e.g., two cues occurring at the same time whenever a particular patient situation or response occurs. Fewer repetitive cues increase task complexity.

Overlapping cues: Cues that are reliable indicators of more than one patient response or situation, e.g., sighing may be a manifestation of shortness of breath or sadness. Overlapping cues increase the complexity of the task (Tanner, 1984, pp. 66–67, citing Hammond, 1966).

Irreducible uncertainty: In some patient states or situations, certainty cannot be achieved—no amount of additional clear thinking, logic, data, or knowledge will reduce the uncertainty (Hammond, 1966, p. 35).

Some cues in the patient situation are both obvious and clear. For example:

A child, seeing the nurse approach with a syringe and needle begins to scream and draws away. In this situation the child's response to anticipated pain is fear.

But not all cues presented by patients and their situations are so easily seen. Some individuals seek to disguise their responses. For example:

Loneliness is the response to a deficit in needed or desired human intimacy. It results in feelings of abandonment, emptiness, dissatisfaction, anxiety and depression. Sullivan wrote that loneliness is so dreaded and painful that it tends to be avoided, disguised or denied (1953). The lonely person could say, "I feel very lonely," a clear and obvious cue. However, loneliness may need to be diagnosed on the basis of more obscure, disguised cues such as:

Symptoms:	Time oriented complaints: "The days and nights are long." "I hate weekends."
	"I do not see the family or friends much. They are very busy you know."
Signs:	A change in usual pace of activities, e.g., from being busy to sitting back and doing little or the reverse.
	Changes in amount of talking, i.e., more or less.
	Less attentiveness to others.
	Reports of more physical symptoms, increased visits to the doctor, and efforts to prolong visits.
	Inability to concentrate—flitting from one activity to another.
	Avoiding decisions.
	Increased irritability (Carnevali, 1986).

In this human response, manifestations often are disguised and unclear.

Nurses diagnose many phenomena in which cues may be given in a very subtle way or may be quite disguised, e.g., fear or anxiety may be manifested as anger. Lack of clarity in cues contributes to complexity in diagnosis.

Probabilities

Clinical judgments about nursing diagnosis and prognosis are based upon the expectation that certain cues or cue clusters are associated with particular diagnoses. In 1988 criteria for major and minor characteristics were set by NANDA for validation studies of proposed nursing diagnoses. The difference is the empirical difference in the percent of cases in which the characteristic is to be found in a given diagnostic category. The percentages are:

Major: present in 80–100% of cases

Minor: present in 50–79% of cases

Extensive validation studies have not yet been done on a variety of diagnoses accepted for clinical testing. Another approach is that of seeking consensus based on the experience of expert clinicians. Carpenito (1989) has used this strategy and set "must be present" (100%) as the criterion for major characteristics (Carpenito, 1989, p. 16).

Diagnostic task complexity is based in part upon the uncertainty that cues and cue clusters are reliably associated with a given diagnosis. That uncertainty can be reduced by the accumulation of cues in which each one has been associated with the diagnosis, thus increasing the probability that the diagnosis is a valid one. At the same time, knowledge of the range of variability in manifestations is also important.

See *Exercise Set 9* for activities to explore levels of complexity in the diagnostic task.

Summary

Many factors influence nurses' effectiveness and efficiency as diagnosticians. Some of these are intrapersonal—one's education and experience; one's beliefs about the nature of nursing and clinical judgments, including the nature of one's involvement with patients and families; one's sensory and cognitive capacities and emotional status. Some factors are interpersonal—nature of the clientele; length and duration of contact with them; attitudes of one's colleagues in nursing, medicine and other health care disciplines; role expectations; job descriptions; and feedback. Some factors emerge from the work environment—type of health care service provided, institutional philosophy, space, privacy, job requirements, caseloads, and technology. Finally, clinical judgment is affected by the nature of the diagnostic task itself.

It is wise occasionally to "take an inventory" of factors shaping one's current diagnostic capabilities and examine their potential for enhancing or reducing diagnostic effectiveness. Where it is possible to modify the factors to improve one's diagnostic capacities, action can be taken. When it is not possible to make changes, at least one's awareness can be heightened to try to use positive factors to enhance one's skill and to minimize harmful biases or effects on one's diagnosing.

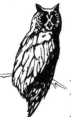

Exercises on Factors Affecting Clinical Judgment and Decision Making

Set 1 □ *Discipline Influence on Diagnostic Perspective*

1. Select a patient situation in which a variety of health care disciplines currently contribute to that person's health care. Concretely identify the nursing focus, nursing diagnoses, and treatment plan for yourself. Then, interact with students or professionals in the other disciplines involved, e.g., pharmacy, nutrition, social work, medicine. Ask them to describe the case and identify their discipline's focus, any problem areas they have identified, and treatment activities

they have planned. Contrast it with your own. Share your diagnoses and treatment plans and seek their reactions. Consider how their input affects your diagnoses and treatment plan. Consider also how your nursing data, diagnoses, and treatment plans should affect those of the other health care providers.

2. Present the same case to nurses with different specialty areas and ask what problem areas they would identify and how they would treat them.

3. Examine the limitations each one brought and the richness of perspective when their discipline-specific perceptions and expertise were added to your own. Did you sense any areas where there would be difficulties in integrating either diagnoses or treatments?

Set 2 □ Influence of Formal and Informal Role Expectations on Diagnosis and Treatment Planning

1. Identify the formal role expectations with regard to nursing diagnosis and treatment planning that are **overtly** held on the nursing unit where you currently provide care. Describe how these formal role expectations are specifically communicated.

2. Identify the nurse coordinator's and staff nurses' **informal** role expectations about the value and priority of nursing diagnosis and treatment planning and what constitutes excellence in these nursing tasks. Observe and identify specifically how these are communicated verbally, in actions, in attitudes, in priorities. (There may be a wide range of expectations and valuing as well as both overt and subtle signals—try to identify them.)

3. Identify your personal role expectations about the value and priority you believe you assign to nursing diagnosis and treatment planning in your professional life (be honest with yourself). Identify your actions, words, and behavior that enabled you to make these judgments about yourself. What behavior (verbal, nonverbal, actions) do you believe you engage in that communicates your values and role expectations to other nursing colleagues.

4. Take a formal nursing history on a patient to whom you will give care. Then as you continue to encounter the patient and the family, interact in ways that enable you to really come to "know" what the health situation means to each of them and the ways in which they are responding (physiologically, psychologically, socially). Contrast what you are learning on an ongoing basis with what you learned in the initial encounter. How do they differ? What contribution does each one make?

Set 3 □ Influence of Other Professional Groups on Nurses' Diagnostic and Treatment Planning Behavior

1. Observe and describe the reactions and behavior of physicians to nursing diagnoses and treatment plans communicated to them orally or in writing. Ask physicians their reactions to nurses' diagnoses and treatment plans. Consider how these responses tend to influence your behavior in diagnosing and planning

care and in communicating these judgments and decisions to individual physicians. Ask other nurses on the unit if or how physician reactions to nursing diagnoses and treatment plans influence their activities in these areas.

2. Discuss with members of other health care disciplines, e.g., physical therapists, occupational therapists, speech therapists, nutritionists, social workers who give direct care to patients on your unit what their professional reactions are to nurses' diagnoses and treatment plans. How does this influence the way in which you/other nurses communicate your care plans to them?

3. Which accrediting agencies are involved in auditing documentation of care in your institution? Read the part of the accreditation regulations having to do with nursing documentation. How do the regulations and the predicted behavior of accreditors influence diagnosing and treatment planning behavior and documentation on your unit? In which ways is it seen as a positive influence? As a negative influence?

4. Are there any legal guidelines in the institution that affect what you document and the language you are expected to use?

Set 4 □ Influence on Diagnosis of Dealing with a Specialized Clientele

1. Talk with nurses who work in different clinical specialty areas and who care for clientele of different ages. Ask them about high frequency, high priority nursing (not medical) problems they tend to look for among their patients and families. Contrast your findings and consider the higher expertise in some diagnostic areas and treatment planning and lower expertise in others.

2. Consider your own clinical practice. What diagnostic areas are you prepared to notice among your patients? Which areas do you feel especially well prepared to diagnose and treat? Are there areas that you consider less often? not at all? where you feel lacking in expertise? What implications does this have for your practice?

Set 5 □ Influence of Equipment on Nursing Diagnosis

1. Identify the equipment or findings from equipment (e.g., computers, CAT scans, MRI, EEGs, EKGs, laboratory tests, pathology reports, x-ray readings) that are routinely available for patients on your unit. Identify specific ways in which they influence nursing diagnosis and treatment planning.

2. Role-play a situation in which you are a consulting telephone nurse in a Health maintenance Organization or a pediatric poison control center. Ask a classmate or friend to enact the person to call you on the telephone and to take on the voice, language, audible signs and symptoms of the person being enacted. Notice the strategies you use to enable the "patient" to provide the information you need to make clinical judgments—both medical and nursing. What strategies could you engage in to come to "know" the patient and communicate this concern and caring during a telephone encounter?

Set 6 □ Influence of Forms on Nursing Diagnosis

1. Examine the forms used for documenting the nursing database and for nursing diagnosis and treatment planning. What aspects of the patient's response and situation receive high priority? Low priority? Are not considered? Are there areas you wish were omitted? Are there some that you wish were included that are not on the forms? Give a rationale for your answers.
2. Identify ways in which the structure of the forms influences nurses' freedom or constraints in data collection, diagnosing, and treatment planning?
3. Do you see many nursing diagnoses that are almost the same for patients on your unit? Do you see individualized, specific, diverse diagnoses?
4. Are standard treatment plans used on your unit? Without modification? Individualized for each patient?
5. Are there diagnoses and treatment plans that emerge from you or other nurses as a result of really coming to "know" the patient or family?

Set 7 □ Influence of Patient Assignment on Diagnostic Behavior

1. Identify the assignment pattern on your nursing unit. Do nurses tend to have responsibility for diagnosing and planning nursing care for the same patients from admission to discharge or over a designated period of time? on readmission or in return visits to a clinic? Is responsibility for diagnosis and treatment associated with a caseload that is unpredictable from day to day? Is one nurse assigned to do all the admission nursing assessments?
2. Talk with nurses about how patient assignment affects their sense of responsibility for making nursing diagnoses and planning patient care; their actual activities; their valuing of the activities.

Set 8 □ Characteristics of the Diagnostician and Effect on Diagnosis

1. Examine the skills and characteristics identified in the section on "Characteristics of the Individual Diagnostician" pp. 158–159. Ask your watchbird to help you to identify your current assets. Identify areas where growth or change is needed in order to improve your diagnostic effectiveness. Observe both long term characteristics and current factors in other nurses to see if you can link them to the documented nursing assessments, diagnoses, and treatment plans.

Set 9 □ Influence of the Diagnostic Task on Diagnosis

1. Examine the cue characteristics on p. 160. Then do a nursing assessment on a patient. After you have completed the assessment, again look at the cue characteristics. Using the characteristics of cues (number, reliability, redundancy, overlapping, irreducible uncertainty), describe the cues in the patient situation you just assessed. Then identify how the cue characteristics in this situation affect the ease or difficulty of making a diagnosis. Did you sense any disguised or muted

cues? Was any part of the patient's situation or response one where there was a risk of disguised cues?

2. If your clinical situation permits, seek to encounter a patient who is having newly experienced acute pain and collect the cues associated with response to that pain. Cues you may see include: *physiological*—pallor, increases in blood pressure, pulse, respirations, muscle spasms, sweating, pupil dilation; inability to concentrate; *body language*—guarding, tense body position, holding, rubbing or pulling at a body part, grimacing, writhing; *verbal expressions*—complaints or descriptions of pain experience; *nonverbal sounds*—crying, moaning, grunting, screaming. Be as specific in your descriptors as you can.

Seek also to encounter a patient who is suffering from chronic pain, e.g., advancing cancer, and collect cues. Cues you may see include: *physiological*—little or no change associated with the effects of the autonomic system, loss of ability to concentrate, shortened attention span, loss of appetite, fatigue, altered/disturbed sleep patterns, increasing sensitivity to other stimuli (sensory overload) leading to irritability, inability to tolerate criticism, and withdrawal, depression; *body language*—muscle rigidity, bruxing, restless legs, holding tight to someone or something, rubbing the area, putting pressure on the area, immobility, repositioning, reduced activity, facial stillness; *verbal expressions*—more passive, less verbal in describing the pain, underreporting or failing to adequately describe pain (Abrams, 1966), repetitive speech, withdrawal in social interaction; *nonverbal sounds*—increased silence, moaning, groaning, crying out during sudden increases in pain (Carnevali and Reiner, 1990, pp. 399–400; Coyle and Foley, 1985). Compare the complexity of the diagnostic task in these two patient situations where pain is a common problem.

References

ABRAMS RD: The patient with cancer: his changing pattern of communication. *New England Journal of Medicine* 274:317, 1966.

BENEDICT S: The suffering associated with lung cancer. *Cancer Nursing* 12:34, 1989.

CARNEVALI D, REINER A: *The Cancer Experience: Nursing Diagnosis and Management.* Philadelphia: J.B. Lippincott, 1990.

CARNEVALI D: Loneliness. In Carnevali D, Patrick M (eds): *Nursing Management for the Elderly.* 2nd ed. Philadelphia: J.B. Lippincott, 1986, pp. 287–298.

CARPENITO L: *Nursing Diagnosis: Application to Clinical Practice.* 4th ed. Philadelphia: J.B. Lippincott, 1991.

COYLE N, FOLEY K: Pain in patients with cancer: profile of patients and common pain syndromes. *Seminar in Oncology Nursing* 1:93, 1985.

DUCLOW D: Into the whirlwind of suffering: Resistance and transformation. *Second Opinion* 9:10, 1988.

FELDMAN H: Pain. In Patrick M, Woods S, Craven R, Rokosky J, Bruno P (eds): *Medical-

Surgical Nursing: Pathophysiological Concepts. 2nd ed. Philadelphia: J.B. Lippincott, 1991.

Fox RC: The evolution of medical uncertainty. *Millbank Memorial Fund Quarterly: Health and Society* 58(1):1–49, 1980.

GOODMAN M: Delivery of cancer chemotherapy. In Burd S, McCorkle R, Grant M (eds): *Cancer Nursing: A Comprehensive Textbook.* Philadelphia: J.B. Lippincott, 1991, pp. 291–320.

HAMMOND K: Clinical inference in nursing: II. A psychologist's viewpoint. *Nursing Research* 15:27–38, 1966.

JOY M, POLLARD C, NUNAN T: Diurnal variation in exercise in angina pectoris. *British Heart Journal* 48:156–160, 1982.

LEE K: Nursing care of patients with disturbances in arousal and sleep patterns. In Patrick M, Woods S, Craven R, Rokosky J, Bruno P (eds): *Medical-Surgical Nursing: Pathophysiological Concepts,* 2nd ed. Philadelphia: J.B. Lippincott, 1991, pp. 79–91.

LEMMER B: Circadian rhythms in the cardiovascular system. In Arendt J, Minors D, Waterhous J (eds): *Biological Rhythms in Clinical Practice.* London: Wright, 1989, pp. 51–70.

MISHEL M: Uncertainty in illness. *Image: Journal of Nursing Scholarship* 20:225, 1988.

MULLER J, LUDMER P, WILLICK S, TOFFLER G, AYLMER G, KLANGOS I, STONE P: Circadian variation in the frequency of sudden cardiac death. *Circulation* 75(1):131–138, 1987.

PEPLAU H: A working definition of anxiety. In Burd S, Marshall M (eds.): *Some Clinical Approaches to Psychiatric Nursing.* New York: Macmillian, 1963.

PRESCOTT P, BOWEN S: Physician-nurse relationships. *Annals of Internal Medicine* 103:127–133, 1985.

PRESCOTT P, DENNIS K, JACOX A: Clinical decision making of staff nurses. *Image: Journal of Nursing Scholarship* 19(2):56–62, 1987.

RHODES V, WATSON P, JOHNSON M: Association of chemotherapy-related nausea and vomiting with pretreatment and posttreatment anxiety. *Oncology Nursing Forum* 13:41, 1986.

STEIN L, WATTS D, HOWELL T: The doctor-nurse game revisited. *New England Journal of Medicine* 322(8):546–549, 1990.

STEIN L: The doctor-nurse game. *Archives of General Psychiatry* 16:699–703, 1967.

SULLIVAN HS: *The Interpersonal Theory of Psychiatry.* New York: W.W. Norton, 1953.

TANNER C: Factors affecting the diagnostic process. In Carnevali D, Mitchell P, Woods N, Tanner C (eds): *Diagnostic Reasoning in Nursing.* Philadelphia: J.B. Lippincott, 1984.

TANNER C, BENNER P, CHESLA C, GORDON D: The phenomenology of knowing the patient. Submitted for publication.

WHITLEY G: Anxiety (Mild, Moderate, Severe, Extreme/Panic). In McFarland G, Thomas M: *Psychiatric Mental Health Nursing: Application of the Nursing Process.* Philadelphia: J.B. Lippincott, 1991, pp. 145–152.

WILLIAMS B, KARLS J, WANDREI K: The Person-in-Environment (PIE) system for describing problems of social functioning. *Hospital and Community Psychiatry* 40(11):1125–1127, 1989.

7

Organizing Knowledge for Diagnostic and Treatment Decisions

Throughout all of the cognitive processes involved in making diagnostic and prognostic judgments and treatment decisions, knowledge and experience are drawn to working memory from long term memory. Without knowledge and examples from long term memory it would be impossible to recognize and interpret the stimuli, consider diagnoses, make prognostic judgments, or generate therapeutic treatment decisions.

Diagnostic Reasoning in the Real World of Nursing Practice

In the world of nursing practice, clinical judgments and decisions usually are not made in quiet, calm settings with ample time for deliberation. Instead, they are made in busy, pressure-filled clinical settings. Nurses have heavy caseloads. In acute care settings (where two-thirds of all nurses work), patient turnover is usually rapid, patients are acutely ill, and medical care with its high technology tends to commandeer nurses' attention. The nurses' station and entire clinical unit bustle with competing demands and distractions. Patient or family problems with the health experience often emerge quickly and require immediate diagnosis and treatment decisions. Additionally, while many patient health problems have recognizable commonalities, there can be many subtle individualizing features, creating the need for individualized, specific diagnosis and treatment decisions. Ambulatory care clinics present the same hectic environment and pace. In long term care settings, changes in patients tend to be slower (often not easily noticed), creating a different form of diagnostic difficulty. In addition, case loads tend to be larger, leaving less time to spend with each person. Case loads in home care are also heavy and diagnoses complex. Treatment plans, often involving the mobilization and maintenance of external resources, are difficult and time consuming.

All this suggests that it is not enough for nurses to acquire the knowledge base needed for their practice. In addition, the theoretical and clinical knowledge as well as patient experiences need to be stored in such a manner that they are retrievable when they are required, even under adverse working conditions.

Activities Involving Long Term Memory in Clinical Practice

Long term memory, as it is used in clinical nursing practice, may be likened to a filing system. It needs to accommodate three functions:

- storage of new knowledge and experiences;
- modification of material already stored; and
- retrieval of stored material when it is needed.

Storage of New Knowledge and Clinical Experiences

New knowledge and experiences need to be stored for subsequent retrieval. In long term memory, little information is thought to be lost; however, it is not always easy to gain access to what is stored there.

Nurses engaging in nursing diagnosis, prognostic judgments, and treatment decisions need to feel confident about being able to gain access to relevant knowledge and patient instances as quickly as the presenting clinical situation demands. This suggests that some consistent structure should be used to store material in long term memory. Such structure could facilitate both the storing and retrieval of information.

Modification of Previously Stored Material

In the course of nurses' clinical practice, previously "known" and stored knowledge is constantly being modified by new information and experiences. If knowledge was stored earlier in a haphazard, disorganized pattern, it could be more difficult to modify existing diagnostic concepts. One might merely add new knowledge into a jumble of preexisting information and experience. On the other hand, if commonly used diagnostic, prognostic, and treatment concepts are stored in a more orderly fashion, it may be possible instead to attach new knowledge and experience to existing material in an effective way.

Retrieval of Knowledge and Clinical Instances When Needed

The major purpose for storage of knowledge and clinical experience is to have access to them when the clinical situation calls for it. Sometimes the demand for knowledge and previous clinical instances is urgent—a patient's life or well-being depends on immediate access as a basis for almost instantaneous nursing judgment and actions. At other times, a patient or family situation is highly ambiguous or complex, and there is a need to gain access over time to multiple diagnostic clusters and patient instances as a basis for understanding what is being observed. The system used to store diagnostic and treatment concepts, the patient instances, and the linkages between them should accommodate effectiveness in both the rapid judgment and action requirements of the emergency situation and the slower, complex deliberations of other situations.

Creating One's Library of Diagnostic Concepts

Organizing one's knowledge of diagnostic-treatment concepts and the linkages between them is an activity individual diagnosticians must do for themselves. Others may offer a structure and knowledge, and clinical practice provides clinical knowledge and patient instances. However, development of one's own structure and system for nursing knowledge and experience and the actual storage of knowledge and experience is a personal activity. No one can do it for another person.

Each person's professional knowledge base is built with or without awareness in each theory or laboratory class, in each day of professional practice, and in each patient or family encounter.

There are many ways to store one's body of nursing knowledge in long term memory. Some nurses treat professional long term memory like a "junk drawer." They allow knowledge and experiences to fall in with little deliberate processing or organization. It is possible to locate and retrieve what is in the junk drawer, but it can be inefficient, particularly when the need to make judgments and decisions is urgent and the clinical environment is hectic.

A more systematic way of looking at storing knowledge and experience in long term memory might be to liken it to a cerebral "library." This library contains "books" on particular diagnostic/prognostic/treatment concepts and "videos" of related clinical experiences. A system of linkages among them permits the diagnostician to "check out" related diagnostic/treatment concepts and patient instances as needed. In this cerebral library, some books will be large, some small, depending on the current level of knowledge and experience. Some subjects will have multiple videos of examplar patient instances with varying scenarios, and other subjects will have only a few or none. Most diagnostic concepts will contain both theory and experience, but some will contain only one. For example:

> A student who has had theory courses in psychology and pathophysiology but no clinical experience in care of patients receiving chemotherapy could have a "book" containing knowledge about role theory and family theory as well as effects of chemotherapy on malignancies and on the body. However, the related library of experiential "videos" awaits actual experiences. Patient instances (videos) of seeing effective and ineffective family coping with a mother's fluctuating capacities to maintain her maternal and spousal roles would come in encountering or learning about patients and families who are facing these challenges and who respond in varying ways.

The beginning student's nursing library tends to be a small one. It grows with more course work and clinical experience. Discipline-specific course work tends to lend perspective and structure as well as knowledge to the library. Many nursing curricula are structured in accordance with a particular conceptual framework resulting in a tendency for students experiencing that curriculum to organize their "memory libraries" with a congruent structure.

An experienced clinician tends to develop both a general library and a specialized one. When a nurse specializes in one field or one type of clientele, obviously there are more and bigger books devoted to diagnostic concepts in this area as well as greater depth. Similarly, the video library of patient instances in a specialty area probably will be large and will contain exemplars featuring both commonalities and wide variability. Over time, as the clinical specialist develops certain parts of the cerebral library, other parts may receive less attention. "Books and videos" in unused parts of the memory library could become out of date. Many nurses who specialize are aware of their areas of high expertise and their lack of updated "books and patient videos" in other areas. They consult others when their libraries are lacking in sufficient current books and videos to adequately address patients' and families' problems.

Overall Structure of Discipline-specific "Libraries" in Long Term Memory

Each health care discipline brings to its clinical practice a somewhat different perspective and knowledge base. Therefore, it stands to reason that professionals in their respective fields will have a different body of knowledge and patient instances to store in long term memory. There will also be a different structure or category system for storing content. Pharmacists' knowledge base and patient instances will have a different focus than that of nurses. The structure of a pharmacist's memory library will be different from that of a nurse, a dentist, or a physical therapist. The overall structure of one's memory library should enhance storage and retrieval of professionally needed knowledge and experience.

Within the nursing profession the prevailing and officially approved structure is based on human responses to actual and potential health situations. The nine NANDA categories of human responses, defined in Appendix A p. 233, typify this structure. Another commonly used structure for human responses is Gordon's 11 functional health patterns shown in Appendix C.

A model that integrates functioning with the contextual demands of daily living placed on the functional capacities and external resources is found in Carnevali's "Daily Living ↔ Functional Health Status Model," described in Appendix D. These are samples of commonly used structures for nurse's knowledge and patient instances in the long term memory library. Other nursing theoretical frameworks used by nurses as a way of structuring their nursing library include: adaptation (Roy and Robert, 1981) and self-care (Orem, 1985).

A Structure for Organizing Diagnostic Concepts

Not only can one develop an overall structure for one's discipline-specific memory library, it is also efficient to develop a consistent system or organization for content within diagnostic concepts—the "books" and "videos." Then, no matter which diagnostic concept is retrieved, the content structure is dependably consistent. And, whenever one needs to store new information, places for storing it are also constant.

One system that has been found to be workable and useful is offered in this chapter.[1] An overview is shown in Display 7-1. Each of the headings is discussed in more detail in the following pages.

Title

Each diagnostic concept "book" needs a **title** that clearly labels the diagnostic concept. Some will have general titles, such as "Impaired Verbal Communication." Others will have quite specific titles, such as "Impaired Communication with Parkinsonian Facial Immobility."

Patient instance "videos," stored in episodic memory, might be grouped under general category titles such as: "Parkinsonian Facial Immobility" and "Impaired Communication." Then, various experiences with patients having Parkinson's disease and facial immobility, in which communication became a problem to the patient or others, could be stored, e.g., Joe and his wife; Rose and her sister; John and his caregiver; Sarah and her children.

Beyond having a title for retrieval, some patient instances stored in long term memory may have no additional structure; others may be further categorized for memorability in terms of particular features. Diagnostic concept "books," however, usually will have additional structure.

The Nature of the Phenomenon or Situation

Obviously, the first content to be addressed in one's diagnostic concept book is a description of the phenomenon or situation to be diagnosed. For example:

Fatigue: Fatigue . . . a personally experienced state and sensation . . . a normal transient response of sensations of tiredness associated with the expenditure of energy . . . a prolonged state of inadequate energy that can create problems in managing the requirements of daily living . . . a symptom associated with many forms of pathology and medical treatment.

---

[1] See Carnevali D, Reiner A: *The Cancer Experience: Nursing Diagnosis and Management*, Philadelphia: J.B. Lippincott, 1990, for examples of nursing knowledge about a variety of common human responses to both health maintenance and the illness experience organized using this consistent structure.

DISPLAY 7-1
OUTLINE FOR ORGANIZATION OF CONTENT IN DIAGNOSTIC
AND TREATMENT CONCEPTS

Nature of Phenomenon or Situation

Description of problem area and elements in it

Underlying Mechanisms

Description of factors that effect changes in functioning or daily living from the
perspectives of:

Pathophysiology and factors related to medical treatment. Includes
pathologies and effects of all medical diagnostic and treatment activities
on functional capacities and daily living.

Areas of daily living affecting and affected by phenomenon (varies with phenomenon). Includes activities in daily living, events in daily living (personal, health-related), demands in daily living (self-expectations, demands
of others and of possessions), environmental features in either institutional
or home and community setting, and values and beliefs.

Areas of functional health status affecting and affected by the phenomenon.
Varies with phenomenon but often includes strength and endurance for
physical, emotional, and intellectual work; cognition; motivation;
courage; communication; and mood.

Nursing Diagnosis and Treatment

Diagnostic Targets

Focus for assessment and diagnosis. Targets always include patients and their
presenting situation. Other frequent diagnostic targets include critical family
members, companions, caregivers, co-workers, or sexual partners, when these
individuals have an impact on patient's well-being.

Risk Factors

Cues in presenting situation that suggest higher potential for occurrence of
problems in daily living, dysfunction, inadequate capacity to manage the requirements of daily living, or deficits in external resources.

Diagnostic Areas

Specific diagnostic categories that identify problem areas and related factors.
They focus on daily living, areas of dysfunction, or status of resources that
impairs effective management of daily living in the presenting situation.

Manifestations

Signs and symptoms that tend to be associated with the phenomenon identified in the diagnostic area; findings that give evidence that daily living is adversely affecting the situation or that deficits in functioning or external resources interfere with effective management of daily living. (Note: Data on strengths in patterns of daily living, functional capacity, and external resources are used as a means of ruling out problems and as elements in decisions about treatment strategies.)

Prognostic Variables

Variables that predict the course of events, trajectory, and outcome in the diagnosed problem areas and the likelihood of satisfaction with the resultant quality of life.

Complications

Sequelae associated with failure to manage daily living, functioning, or external resources effectively; iatrogenic effects of particular nursing interventions.

Treatment Guidelines

Strategies prescribed to help the patient, family, or others modify daily living or their functional capacity or use their external resources in such a way as to promote more effective and satisfying daily living.

Evaluation

Variables in which data are collected on an ongoing basis to measure changes in daily living (in any of the relevant subcategories), in functioning, or in availability or use of external resources.

Adapted from Carnevali D, Reiner A: *The Cancer Experience: Nursing Diagnosis and Management.* Philadelphia: J.B. Lippincott, 1990, pp. 16–17.

fatigue level can range from mild lassitude or weariness to total exhaustion and prostration . . . it can be a steady state or fluctuate in predictable or unpredictable patterns.

daily living can increase fatigue when the demands of self, or other-imposed role responsibilities exceed current and projected energy levels, when environmental/architectural features require more energy expenditures, when there is lack of personal and physical support in terms of services and people . . .

fatigue can affect daily living in areas such as tasks requiring physical strength and stamina, cognitive tasks, interpersonal relationships, and adjustments that must be made to bring requirements into line with energy levels (Carnevali and Reiner, 1990, pp. 178–179).

Asthenia: Asthenia . . . personally experienced ongoing state of serious mental and physical fatigue plus generalized and progressive weakness (Bruerra and MacDonald, 1988) . . .

progressively erodes capacity to independently manage the requirements of daily living . . . creates new challenges for patients, caregivers, and family members (Carnevali and Reiner, 1990).

Note that the descriptions address the phenomenon from a nursing perspective, not that of other disciplines. These are one's nursing diagnostic concept books and videos, not those of the medical domain. A practicing nurse will also have a library of medical concepts closely linked to related nursing concepts. For example, both fatigue and asthenia can be closely linked to medical concepts of cancer (Theologides, 1982; 1986), cancer treatment (Rhoten, 1982; Piper et al., 1987; Haylock and Hart, 1979), major depression congestive heart failure, adrenal insufficiency, endocrine disorders (Patrick et al. 1991). In the medical concept, states of fatigue or asthenia are linked to pathology and response to medical treatment. In the nursing library they focus on human responses in the health-illness experience, problems in functioning, and managing the requirements of daily living and associated external resources as these are linked to pathology and medical treatment.

Underlying Mechanisms

Some knowledge of the phenomenon's underlying mechanisms is essential to understanding linkages with risk factors, manifestations, prognosis, ways in which nursing treatment can affect the variables, and criteria for evaluation of response to treatment. In the earliest clinical encounters with a phenomenon, the "chapter" in the diagnostic concept having to do with underlying mechanisms tends to be used in a very conscious, detailed, and sometimes laborious fashion (Schmidt, Norman, and Boshuizen, 1990). However, with increased familiarity with a given phenomenon, recall of underlying mechanisms is reduced to background knowledge. Its critical elements are threaded through clinical judgments and decisions without as much awareness. The whole of the knowledge is there, but only its important parts are used.

In the nursing domain, the topic of underlying mechanisms is a description of factors linked to changes in functioning, daily living, or external resources. The factors creating these changes may include:

■ Pathophysiology and responses to medical diagnostic and treatment activities, normal age-related factors and status of developmental task achievement.
■ Daily living that creates or affects the phenomenon (activities, events, demands, environment, values, and beliefs).
■ Functional capacities affecting or affected by the phenomenon.
■ Elements of external resources that can affect the phenomenon or situation.

Using the phenomenon of *cancer-related fatigue,* an excerpt from *The Cancer Experience: Nursing Diagnosis and Management* (Carnevali and Reiner, 1990, pp.

179–183 with permission) illustrates content that could be included in underlying mechanisms and the use of structural subcategories.[2]

UNDERLYING MECHANISMS

Pathophysiologic and Iatrogenic Factors

The pathophysiologic factors that underlie fatigue in cancer are complex, interactive, and currently poorly understood. Fatigue frequently precedes and accompanies the diagnosed presence of malignant neoplasia (Theologides, 1982). It accompanies all of the cancer therapies.

Tumor-Related Factors

Malignant neoplasms can cause:

Metabolites (lactate, hydrogen ions, and end products of cell destruction) to accumulate.

Marked increases in Cori cycle activity (anaerobic gluconeogenesis that uses more than normal amounts of energy and produces more lactate).

Muscle force to be impeded by the hydrogen ions produced as lactate accumulates.

Degradation of skeletal muscle related to protein imbalances, caused by altered protein metabolism, protein losses, and tumor need for increased glucose.

Increased metabolic rate as growing tumors burn more calories.

Altered neurotransmission and force of muscle contractions. This occurs with fluid and electrolyte abnormalities, which are associated with the disease process and nutritional deficits.

Changes in oxygenation and reduced oxygen carrying capacity of the blood when hemoglobin drops to low levels.

Fluid and electrolyte imbalances, hypercalcemia, hyperuricemia, hyponatremia, and hypokalemia. These occur with particular tumors and alter neurotransmission and muscle contractions (see above).

Other manifestations associated with the cancer that may compound fatigue include nausea and vomiting, diarrhea, pain, dyspnea, muscle spasms, and itching. Sleep disruption may contribute to fatigue.

---

[2]Citations of the knowledge sources shown in the original text are omitted. It is not likely they would be retained in long term memory as a part of the diagnostic concept of the average practicing nurse.

Anxiety, hopelessness, and grief can affect energy levels, just as lower energy levels can, in turn, depress psychologic responses.

Sensory underload from home and treatment setting environments as well as changes in the person's mobility can create inadequate sensory stimulation of the reticular activating system. One manifestation of this reduced stimulation can be fatigue.

Diagnostic Tests

Persons who undergo medical diagnostic testing during the active treatment stage encounter activities and stressors that engender fatigue through disruption of eating and elimination patterns in preparation for tests as well as through the discomforts of the actual procedures. News that the response to treatment is not encouraging can cause feelings of increased anxiety or depression, which further engender fatigue.

Surgery

Many aspects of surgery may be synergistic in producing fatigue. These include sedation, anesthesia, decreased ventilation, inadequate normal sleep cycles, analgesia, restricted nutrition and mobility, the physical trauma produced by the surgery itself, plus the continuing effects of underlying disease before and after the surgery.

Chemotherapy

Fatigue is a major iatrogenic effect associated with chemotherapy. Cell destruction end products, nausea, and vomiting are thought to be contributors. Drugs that cross the blood–brain barrier and those that have neurotoxic properties may affect neurotransmission and thus produce fatigue.

Radiation

Fatigue is also a major problem with radiation. The specific mechanism is not known, but possible explanations are the accumulation of cell destruction end products together with the increased metabolic rate needed to dispose of them, toxic metabolites that inhibit cell functioning, anemia from the shortened life of erythrocytes, or the body's mechanism to slow down activity in order to conserve energy. Another factor compounding fatigue may be the energy demands involved in making the daily trip to the health care setting for the treatments over a period of 4 to 5 weeks.

Biologic Response Modifiers

Biologic response modifiers have fatigue as a consistent side effect. The fatigue is not dose dependent, but is cumulative and is sufficient to affect the capacity of the individual to carry out activities of daily living.

Daily Living Factors

Any degree of energy deficit affects the managing of requirements of daily living. Conversely, many aspects of the activities, events, and demands in daily living, as well as barriers in the institutional or home environment, can create demands on already compromised energy levels. When fatigue is extreme the external resources of people and services become crucial to effective management of daily living. The perspective on the patient's daily living thus also involves concern about the daily living and status of support figures—their interest, availability, and physical and emotional capacities, their staying power in the valley times as well as in the good times.

Activities in Daily Living	Physically demanding activities in daily living, mental activities requiring concentration (e.g., balancing the checkbook, filling out the income tax, and preparing shopping lists), and emotion-laden activities (e.g., interaction with family members or health care providers and social situations) that may be stressful are all areas for nursing assessment when energy is low.
Events in Daily Living	Events in daily living that consume energy and can contribute to fatigue include:

Personal and social events requiring extra energy expenditure for personal grooming, travel, social interaction, food preparation, or eating.

Medical events that physiologically cause further energy depletion; create stress, anxiety, or depression, or require energy expenditure for preparation, waiting, travel, or interaction with multiple health care workers.

Past events whose memories create depression or anxiety (e.g., losses, past chemotherapy experiences).

Anticipation of future events that create stress and anxiety (e.g., waiting for the next bone marrow test to determine the status of cells) or signs of separations or future losses.

Demands in Daily Living	*Self-expectations:* These demands can involve the person's self-requirement to maintain, modify, or relinquish usual patterns of grooming, home maintenance, and family, work, and social role obligations.

Expectations of others: Others may expect the patient to either continue or be released from previous standards, role activities, role behaviors, and relationships. Institutions may demand that the patient be involved in activities that require energy expenditures (e.g., participation in preventive or rehabilitative activities following treatment, or self-care activities such as pulmonary hygiene or ostomy care).

Possessions: Possessions such as pets, car, home, or yard make demands for expenditure of energy.

Environment for Daily Living

The institutional, home, or work environment may generate sensory underload or overload, stressors, or immobilization, thus contributing to fatigue.

The person's environment may compound fatigue by requiring extra expenditure of energy to accomplish activities in daily living (e.g., stairs, distances, lack of facilities or conveniences, and difficult terrain).

Values and Beliefs

Personal values play an important role in managing daily living with fatigue. Some previously held standards for self-care and home maintenance can no longer be maintained because they require energy expenditures beyond one's currently available resources. Previously held and valued social roles, control over lifestyle, and goals that require energy expenditure may all be in jeopardy during cancer treatment.

Societal beliefs that can affect energy expenditure include those dealing with patient obligations to maintain, modify, or relinquish role obligations during illness or treatment. These can be particularly troublesome when no visible signs of illness are present or when energy levels wax and wane over prolonged periods of time during the course of chemotherapy.

Functional Health Status

Functional capacities for meeting the requirements of daily living when fatigue is a problem include physical strength and endurance, cognition, sexuality, and emotions.

Strength and Endurance

Fatigue associated with cancer and its treatment affects one's capacity to engage in physical, mental, and emotional work and one's endurance to meet the required activities in daily living. Difficulties can be identified by balancing the patient's present and predicted energy status, based on pathophysiology, iatrogenic factors, and emotional status, with the identified requirements in the person's daily living in the present and future.

Cognition

Managing daily living with fatigue requires the capacity to understand (at the application level):

The causes of and predicted pattern for fatigue in the presenting situation,

Strategies for managing stressors, sensory environment, activities, demands, and environmental features in order to keep them within the current and predicted energy levels,

The usefulness of noting patterns of high and low energy levels as a basis for planning activities and treatments,

The value to one's morale of investing energy to have at least one valued experience each day,

Strategies for conserving energy within one's particular environment and daily living requirements,

Strategies for mobilizing and maintaining external resources to cover tasks one no longer has the energy to perform,

Interpersonal skills needed to renegotiate roles to make them congruent with current and anticipated levels of energy.

Sexuality

Depressed energy in the absence of other symptoms can decrease interest in sexual activity. This can, in turn, create stresses between the partners.

Emotions

Functional capacity can be affected by the patient's usual moods of optimism or pessimism in stressful and nonstressful times and by the moods in the present situation.

External Resources for Managing Daily Living With Fatigue

Fatigue can interfere with meeting even the basic requirements of daily living. Therefore, the status of availability, acceptability, and usability of external resources in the forms of people and services is an important consideration.

People

The availability of others to assist the patient may be determined by asking:

What support persons are available?

What is the status of their physical and emotional strength and endurance?

Do they have a working knowledge of helping strategies in the presenting situation?

Services

Support services may be assessed with the following questions:

Are transportation and other energy-conserving services available, and does the person have sufficient financial resources to purchase these services?

> What types of services will the patient and family accept?

It is obvious that all of this knowledge could not be retrieved into working memory's 5 to 9 chunk capacity each time a nurse sees a person trying to meet the requirements of daily living in the presence of fatigue. However, a brief outline of salient points could permit the nurse to remember that:

> In cancer, both the tumor and any of the treatments produce by-products that create a physiologic basis for prolonged, serious fatigue.

> In daily life, fatigue will affect capacity to meet requirements in the areas of activities, events, self-expectations and demands of others, environmental features and values (personal priorities and societal beliefs about the person's role obligations).

> Priority functional areas to consider include strength and endurance, cognition, emotional responses, and, in some situations, sexuality.

> External resources involving people, services, money and transportation are important considerations.

Thus, four pages have been condensed to four small chunks that can guide the search for patient/caregiver/family/environmental data, diagnostic areas, prognosis, and focus for treatment and evaluation.

Diagnostic Targets

Medicine's diagnosis and treatment focuses primarily on the patient and occasionally on patient contacts where the pathology is contagious. On the other hand, nurses are frequently involved in diagnosing not only the individual but also caregivers, members of the family, sexual partners, or others who closely share the person's health-related experience and daily living. Nurses who work in occupational health, school settings or governmental bureaucracies may be involved in diagnosing patient situations influenced by employers, teachers, classmates, co-workers, or people in bureaucracies. Targets for nursing assessment, diagnosis and treatment will tend to vary with different problem areas. For example, in addition to primary focus on the patient:

- When a problem involves prolonged difficulty in eating, an important target for diagnosis is the food-preparer/caregiver and those who share mealtimes or other eating experiences.
- When a problem involves sensory underload or overload, assessment and diagnosis consider the environment, people and pets involved in creating stimuli in the patient's world.

Where diagnostic focus is primarily on a family or another group, targets for diagnosis and treatment can include other individuals and groups having impact on the family or group's diagnosed problem(s). For example:

- The values, priorities and goals of a family receiving health care from an agency are different enough from those of the care providers that there is an impasse and growing friction. It will not be enough to diagnose and treat the family; judgments and attention will also need to be given to the care provider(s) involved.
- The family's desire and need to know about a prognosis conflicts with the doctor's usual pattern of providing information (the family wishes to know and the doctor is reluctant to share the information; or the family does not wish to know, and it is the physician's pattern to be very open about prognosis).
- A family feels that they have enough data to support commitment of a psychotic member for his own and their safety; the mental health professional disagrees.

It is important to include the diagnostic target(s) as part of the diagnostic concept. While it is true that the nurse may work through the patient or family to influence others, it is important to consider which individuals or systems can have impact on patient or family well-being and to develop plans that will enable the patient or family to deal with them. This means diagnosing the difficulties and making prognostic judgments prior to assisting the patient or family to plan their strategies.

Risk Factors

Risk factors are the characteristics of the person, the antecedent events, or conditions in the situation increasing the likelihood that the phenomenon will occur and that the person(s) involved will experience difficulty in managing it.

Personal Characteristics

Certain personal characteristics tend to foster the probability that a problem will occur. For example:

Older males are more likely to commit suicide than older females.

Individuals whose self-concept and self-esteem are closely linked with being beautiful, having a perfect body, or functioning at a high level in certain areas will have greater difficulty in adjusting to altered appearance or functioning.

Individuals or families who have unrealistic expectations about treatment effects will have greater difficulty in adjusting to outcomes that are incongruent with their expectations.

An individual with an absolute neutrophil count of less than 1,000 is at great risk for infections.

Those who prefer control and power will have difficulty adjusting to situations in which they are dependent.

Those who prefer to live alone will have difficulty in adjusting to congregate living.

Values and beliefs of patient or family that conflict with those of the health care providers will create risks of disagreement, "noncompliance," and emotional distancing of participants.

Antecedent Events

Very often antecedent events create risk factors. For example:

A person who has had negative experiences with health care systems tends to approach subsequent encounters with some pessimism.

An anxious patient whose earlier experience with chemotherapy produced high emetic effects is more likely to have to manage the problems associated with anticipatory nausea and vomiting.

Dysfunctional families tend to break down with the strains associated with new health problems.

A pattern of poor relationships and poor sexual functioning creates risks of difficulties in adjustment if one member has new pathology or iatrogenic effects that alter appearance or sexual capacities.

Earlier drug use can create difficulties in achieving analgesia in subsequent health problems requiring pain control.

Current Conditions

In some situations, current conditions create risks that a problem will occur. For example:

Arrival of a new baby can cause the next older child to regress to less mature behavior.

Living alone is a risk when one may have health-related emergencies or need ongoing care.

A left cerebrovascular accident (CVA) can result in loss of judgment about one's capacity to manage the requirements of daily living, e.g., the person is certain he can manage his finances, drive his car, or live independently, even though his performance indicates that he cannot do any of these things. The risk that there will be conflict between the patient and family members or caregivers is high.

Lack of easy access to toilet facilities can create risk of urinary or fecal incontinence when certain pathology or iatrogenic conditions exist.

Having role obligations that others cannot easily assume increases the risks of difficulties in managing daily living with a variety of symptoms, e.g., fatigue, pain, nausea and vomiting, time for self-care.

Lacking command of language to communicate one's situation or negotiate for meeting one's needs increases the risk for unmet needs.

Lack of predictable, adequate respite can increase the risk of burnout for caregivers having total responsibility for a dependent person.

Living as a child in an abusive home situation creates risks to current and future physical and mental health.

Risk factors associated with different phenomena and situations will be different. For examples of risk factors associated with a variety of phenomena, refer to the risk factor sections throughout *The Cancer Experience: Nursing Diagnosis and Management*. While the content of the book addresses situations linked to neoplastic pathology, the problems are quite generic and can be transposed to many other health-related conditions.

In order to prevent a potential problem, nurses need to be ready to consider risk factors. Then they can be prepared to attend to and identify:

- cues in the person,
- antecedent events, or
- factors in the current situation

that are indicators of potential problems. When nurses sense risk factors in the patient situation, possible problems linked with particular risk factors can be retrieved. The diagnostic reasoning associated with identification of potential problems is the same as that of diagnosing currently existing problems. With *potential problems* the data are in the three categories of risk factors; with *existing problems* they are signs and symptoms—the manifestations.

In addition to being useful in diagnosing potential problems, risk factors can coexist with an already existing problem. Perhaps the risk factors were not recognized early enough or they were so overwhelming that the problem could not be prevented. Then findings on risk factors often turn out to be prognostic variables as well.

Diagnostic Areas

Any phenomenon or general problem area can generate a variety of human responses and situations that require nursing diagnosis and treatment. Note that the content stored in diagnostic concepts are **diagnostic areas**—not diagnoses. Working diagnostic statements include: the specific problem, related factors, and patient responses. They emerge from diagnostic areas but are further refined with the data from the specific patient situation. Diagnostic areas denote broader categories within which specific problems may exist. They are guides to assessment. For example, changes in health status of a family member or an individual often require those involved to make changes involving a diagnostic area of roles and role relationships. The phenomenon or general problem area would be "Altered Role Performance." However, the need to make these changes and the actual changes can spawn a variety of more specific diagnostic possibilities such as:

- Adjustment to specific **disruptions in a role behavior** because of a particular dysfunction, e.g., being a student who moves from being vision impaired to being blind; changing sexual behavior because of becoming HIV positive.

- **Role ambiguity,** e.g., transition from nonpatient to patient status or the reverse, from being healthy to having a chronic disease.
- **Reluctance to accept a change in role** (either loss of a role or taking one on), slowness to move from the sick role because it met the person's need for attention (secondary gain).
- **Role incompetence,** e.g., difficulty in taking on the role of the patient or family member in an informed consent interaction because of deficits in language, courage, or communication skills to negotiate the desired treatment approach.
- **Dissatisfaction with changes in role and role relationships,** e.g., teenage children who, having taken over a parent's home responsibilities during the parent's illness and convalescence, are reluctant to return to the former parent-child relationship; or a patient in treatment whose co-workers attempt to take over aspects of the patient's job that he/she does not wish to relinquish.
- **Lack of negotiating skills to establish a satisfying role and role relationship,** e.g., patient and nurse or other caregiver; a sexual partner with altered functional capacities or attitude.
- **Lack of power to modify an unsatisfactory role or role relationship,** e.g., cancer survivor and prospective employers or insurance companies.
- **Environmental barriers creating difficulties in role relationships,** e.g., isolation precautions, masks, geographic distances to health care settings, lack of privacy in certain health care settings.
- Dealing with **stigmatization** or **being placed in victim/outcast roles,** e.g., a person with autism, positive HIV status, disfigurement with head and neck surgery or burns.
- **Role conflicts** associated with health status and responsibilities or type of health care, e.g., wish for home care instead of institutionalization, wish to discontinue life support systems, desire to work despite physical handicaps, assuming the consumer role in the use of medical services and using medical recommendations for treatments as only one factor in making autonomous choices.

The possible diagnoses associated with any diagnostic area need to be stored with that diagnostic concept "book." They are used in the stage of diagnostic reasoning dealing with retrieval of possible diagnostic explanations and differential diagnosis.

Diagnostic areas are parts of the diagnostic concept "book" that tend to be regularly modified and updated as a result of day-by-day clinical experience and exposure to the thinking of other clinicians in the field. New diagnostic areas are added, current ones may receive added weight because of frequency or significance. Some diagnoses may not be found or may be seen so infrequently that they are relegated to a little used memory area.

Manifestations

Manifestations are the clusters of cues—signs (objective data) and symptoms (subjective data)—associated with a diagnosis. In nursing these signs and symptoms tend to address human responses/functional status, daily living that affects or is affected by the health situation, and availability and use of external resources. Cue clusters are attached to specific diagnostic areas, not just to the general diagnostic category.

Major and Minor Manifestations

Cue clusters are classified in terms of their significance to the diagnosis. Major manifestations are those present in a large proportion of situations where this diagnosis has been made. Minor manifestations may or may not be present and carry less weight (Carpenito, 1989).

Subtle or Disguised Cues

An awareness of the manifestations that might be subtle or disguised is also an important piece of knowledge to be stored as part of the diagnostic concept. Specific characteristics of disguised cues associated with a diagnosis should be stored. For example:

> Chronic pain and loneliness are two states that tend to cause others to distance themselves from a person who has this experience. Individuals who are suffering from pain or loneliness are known to provide cues that are indirect or they disguise and mute their actual experiences.

> In early stages of Alzheimer's disease, individuals may confabulate (fill in gaps in memory with fictitious material) to cover their short term memory losses.

Cues That Should Not Be Present

In addition, the cue cluster may indicate manifestations that should not be present if this diagnosis is to be made. For example:

> A diagnosis of denial of a problem cannot be made if the person recognizes and acknowledges the presence of the specific problem.

> A diagnosis of noncompliance cannot be made if a physiological dysfunction rather than unwillingness deters a person from carrying out a particular task.

> Anxiety is characterized by a nameless threat to personhood, while fear has an identifiable object. If the person can identify the object causing them to feel fearful, one does not make a diagnosis of anxiety.

> A diagnosis of knowledge deficit cannot be accepted if there are findings that the patient-family have the requisite knowledge to manage the health problem but are purposefully not using it because it conflicts with their beliefs or current priorities.

Manifestations of Effective Self-care

Signs and symptoms may also give evidence that problems exist but the individual is currently managing them. This is known as data for ruling out problems that might be expected to exist. For example:

> A teenaged girl has diabetes but may be maintaining a steady blood glucose, monitoring herself consistently, giving her own insulin in a correct pattern, using the exchange diet concept effectively even when eating away from home, and managing developmental tasks in a normal manner.

Including the cue clusters that indicate effective management of specific difficulties is important as nurses seek to diagnose the strengths of health and self-care.

In this area of the diagnostic concept, it is wise also to store information on the nurse's personal beliefs and values as to what constitutes "effective self-management or problem solving." This stored information may be needed when the patient or family are managing problems but perhaps not in the way the nurse would prefer. This is a diagnostic judgment nurses frequently are called on to make—effectiveness as defined by the patient/family or by the nurse.

Prognostic Variables

As discussed in depth in Chapter 4, prognostic variables are indicators of predicted course of events and outcomes associated with a specific diagnosis. The part of the diagnostic concept associated with prognosis involves cues about internal resources, daily living patterns, and external resources that are indicators of the potential for managing the health-related experience and associated requirements of daily living. There are cues or cue clusters that predict positive outcomes and those indicating negative ones, as well as cue clusters suggesting the pattern and rate of change.

At present, the body of nursing knowledge has not specifically identified prognostic variables, so this part of the concept will need to be extrapolated from what literature is available and from clinical experience. Since prognostic judgments are factors important to treatment decisions and evaluations, it is important for nurses and nursing to create and refine the "prognostic chapter" in each diagnostic "book" and "video," even though it has not yet been formalized into nursing thinking.

Complications

Complications are undesired side effects associated with the dynamics of a diagnosed problem or its nursing treatment (iatrogenic).

Complications of the Diagnosed Problem

Complications have long been a part of medical diagnostic concepts but, like prognosis, have not been seen as being applicable to problems in the nursing domain.

However, just as there are complications associated with pathology and its treatment, there are complications associated with human responses to health and illness experiences and difficulties in management of associated daily living. For example:

> An infant, born to a young single mother living below the poverty level and who was abused as a child, is likely to suffer neglect and possible abuse if intervention is not made or is not successful. This is a complication of being born into a particular situation.

> An older person who is demented and vocally disruptive can experience the complication of failure to thrive as family and health care staff withdraw physically and emotionally.

It is important, therefore, that each diagnostic concept contain knowledge about complications with the diagnosed problem itself.

Iatrogenic Complications

Nursing treatment, like medical treatment, can create complications. Failure to act, acting at the wrong time, or engaging in the wrong treatment can create undesired side effects instead of the intended effects. For example:

> Failure to begin and continue consistent range of motion activities shortly after the onset of hemiplegia can result in greater possibility of contractures.

> Failure to give pain medications at an appropriate interval before pain-causing activities or treatment can result in unnecessary suffering or inadequate performance of the activity.

> Use of guilt-producing strategies to try to gain compliance with a health care regimen tends to produce anger, defensiveness, or withdrawal rather than the desired effect.

> Use of restraints to prevent falls and injury can have the iatrogenic effect of causing patients to lose muscle tone and develop contractures making the patient even more vulnerable to falls and injury.

> Use of confrontation as a regular strategy in seeking to gain acknowledgment of a substance abuse problem in a fragile person who is using denial as a defense mechanism can destroy resources rather than build them.

> Use of logic and teaching as a strategy for modifying strongly held beliefs and values tends to be unsuccessful.

> Asking sensitive questions early in an interaction before trust or a logical basis for need-to-know has been established can result in the building of interpersonal barriers rather than openness in communication.

> Teaching about managing requirements of daily living after a myocardial infarc-

tion while the patient is still in the hospital can result in limited learning. If no further teaching takes place, the patient may be functioning without the knowledge needed to be most effective.

Teaching a man with a left CVA about activities in one physical setting and expecting him to be able to transfer this knowledge to other settings is likely to leave him with the capacity to carry out these activities only in the original setting.

Failure to prepare caregivers for the emotional responses that are frequently and normally experienced in providing ongoing care to a dependent person can cause undue suffering if they believe that their feelings of guilt, frustration, and anger are abnormal.

Interrupting normal sleep cycles with monitoring or treatments because of failure to group them or to find out the time when the patient sleeps best can result in sleep deprivation, irritability, fatigue, and even psychosis.

Complications associated with problems in the nursing domain and with nursing treatment are as important as they are in medicine. Since this has not been addressed specifically in nursing literature, it will require some thought and the use of clinical experience to develop these portions of nurses' diagnostic "books."

Treatment Options

The portion of the diagnostic concept devoted to treatment usually requires subheadings to group options for treatment associated with specific diagnostic subcategories. Decisions about what treatments to store in a particular diagnostic subheading will be derived from an understanding of the underlying mechanisms and prognostic data involved with that specific phenomenon or situation. For example:

Nurses who work on head and neck surgery units regularly care for patients whose lips, jaws and swallowing muscles have been radically altered by surgery. Eating and drinking is mechanically difficult. Two frequently occurring diagnostic areas requiring nursing treatment are *grief related to loss of eating competence* and *ineffective individual coping with social/business encounters involving eating.* Treatment will need to address both the grief work and gaining new eating skills and social competencies and be further modified by patient data from the specific situation.

Treatment options can include[3]:

Determine the nature of the specific loss(es) this patient is experiencing. Make a clinical judgment as to the anticipated duration of the losses.

With long-term deficits, determine the degree to which the patient can find

[3]Excerpted with permission from Carnevali D, Reiner A: *The Cancer Experience: Diagnosis and Management.* Philadelphia: J.B. Lippincott 1990, pp. 137-138.

satisfying goals related to eating that are less than a total restitution of previous lifestyle and skills.

If the duration of the dysfunction is limited, emphasize the time-limited nature of the loss (e.g., by marking days off on a calendar).

Indicate the normalcy of the grief being experienced and the legitimacy of grieving behavior: "Of course you are angry (or depressed)—you've had a big loss." Point out that awareness of the normalcy of grief and its stages does not permit escape or minimize the suffering associated with it.

Where losses in eating competence or preferred foods can be improved, offer assistance or resources when the person is able and willing to try them.

Explore the nature of social encounters that are lost or avoided and discuss possibly acceptable alternatives.

Can the person manage to eat dessert in a group setting?

Are there foods that cause fewer problems, so that a menu could be developed that is "safe"?

When new skills of eating have been learned, accompany patient to a "safe" area in the hospital cafeteria or other public place to try out public eating.

Help the patient develop plans and scripts for setting the stage for eating with others or for dealing with any problems that may arise. These should include preparing others for the patient's eating difficulties and offering options (e.g., "I'd like very much to come over for dinner, if you don't mind my bringing my own food—I'm still having difficulty swallowing, so I'm rather limited" or "My eating still isn't very skillful; you may want to wait till I get better at it" or "I couldn't manage a whole meal out, but I'd like very much to join you for dessert" or "My breathing tube (tracheostomy) still makes some noises and I do have to cough at times. I may have to leave the table occasionally so that I won't bother the others. If this is all right with you, I'd enjoy coming.") Some scripts should be developed for the occurrence of sights and sounds that are not usual during social situations (e.g., the sounds or odors from an ostomy, difficulty with food leakage).

Teach the person how to order "safe" foods from a menu or a cafeteria selection, then rehearse. It may be possible to have a supply of typical menus for different types of restaurants available on the unit or in the clinic for this teaching experience.

Explore with the patient who among family and friends are low risk for early practice at eating with others.

Make arrangements for feedback after experiences. Be generous and genuine with praise. Accept difficult experiences as unfortunate, but not unexpected. Diagnose the exact difficulties and help the patient develop alternative strategies and scripts.

On these same units, individuals who will be the caregivers and who will share meals with the patient are also diagnosed and treated. A frequent diagnostic area for caregivers is *potential ineffective individual coping with monotony of preparing the same foods in the same way each day.* Treatment options for this diagnostic area include[4]

> Ask caregiver to identify foods, textures, and food temperatures the patient will accept, then explore other foods with similar tastes, textures, temperatures, and seasonings that might be tried.
>
> Review patient's possible fear of producing additional discomfort or lack of success in eating to prepare caregiver for possible patient reluctance to accept deviations from current diet and eating patterns.
>
> Work out scripts the caregiver can use that encourage but do not appear to "nag" (e.g., "You've had pretty good success with (name the food). I've made some (name the food) that is almost the same, but would give you a little variety. You could try a small bite to see how it goes for you, and if it feels OK you can try a bit more.").

Unlike the previous two sections of prognosis and complications where there is little specific material in the literature, nursing treatment has received greater consideration. There are many books offering research or clinically supported treatment guidelines for a variety of categories of problems in the nursing domain. However, it remains for individual nurses to sift through relevant research and literature to develop the range of treatment options to be stored with particular diagnostic areas. This stored knowledge will be refined by clinical experiences involved in testing and using various treatment options others have recommended so that each treatment activity can be adapted to exactly fit the needs of the patient or family and their situation at the current time.

Evaluation

The final chapter of the diagnostic concept "book" contains information about evaluation. It should include particular areas of functioning, daily living and use of external resources to be evaluated, the kinds and sources of data, the circumstances, timing and duration of data collection, and the standards by which changes in the diagnosed phenomena will be judged. For example,

> If one takes the diagnostic area of eating and swallowing difficulties discussed in the treatment section, the evaluation section of this concept "book" would include:

> Kinds of data: **Subjective data:** reporting of successes and difficulties in retaining foods and liquids in oral cavity, chewing, and swallowing, situations bringing satisfactions and frustrations, residue in mouth after eating; reports on social situa-

---

[4]Excerpted with permission from Carnevali, Reiner, *op. cit.,* p. 141.

	tions attempted and perception of positive and negative aspects.
	Objective data: observation of eating, swallowing competence, leakage of food, residual food in mouth, facial expressions, noises, choking. Condition of skin around mouth, food stains on clothing.
Timing of data collection:	During postoperative hospitalization. In phone contacts, office calls, or home visits in the weeks following discharge. Follow-up calls at intervals dictated by patient and caregiver's progress. Often enough to indicate interest to them but not so often as to seem to be intrusive.
Sources of data:	Patient, caregiver, nurse observer.
Standards:	Degree of success in finding acceptable ways of retaining food and fluids in mouth. Swallows with minimum facial grimacing and choking. Status of skill and satisfaction is use of adaptive devices.
	Range of preferred foods that currently can be successfully ingested.
	Status of development and use of scripts, strategies, and attitudes for handling social situations involving eating difficulties. Degree of comfort and satisfaction.
	Comfort with ordering food from a menu.
	Status of return to a social life that is comparable to the preoperative situation or is comfortable in the postoperative phase.

Evaluation criteria are addressed regularly in nursing literature, although usually in an ideal sense without making adjustments for prognosis. As with all the other sections of the diagnostic concept "book," individual nurses can develop highly refined and creative strategies and criteria for evaluating patient and family response to nursing treatments that include both the ideal desired outcomes and adjustments made for variations in prognoses. The evaluation section of the diagnostic concept may also include forms or schema for accurately and consistently documenting findings.

See *Exercise Sets 1 and 2* for activities on building, modifying and filing diagnostic-treatment concepts in long term memory.

Summary

When a format for storing a diagnostic concept in long term memory is written out as it has been in this chapter, it seems impossibly long and complex. Fortunately, it takes more words to explain about the structure than it does to actually do it. The mind does not need full sentences. Diagnostic concepts can and should be concise as well as systematic. This is not to say that the building of each "book" in one's diagnostic library is not hard work, particularly the first ones.

An easy way to start is with a diagnostic concept that is of particular interest, one that is regularly used so there is ample opportunity for clinical testing. Begin with what you already know, work on it as you have time, sleep on the ideas, think about it when you are not at work, add to it, and revise it. Use it in clinical practice. Discuss it with colleagues. When it begins to take shape and it is possible to see some "holes," consult the literature for specific information to fill these in and also to validate contents. When the first "book" becomes tiresome or boring, move on to another one. See how much easier it gets with practice. (See Exercises at end of chapter for additional guides.)

While it may seem like work to organize one's existing diagnostic concepts in a systematic way and then to add new ones, it is also a form of professional excitement. The journey to diagnostic excellence never ends. There are new insights, new experiences and new knowledge to be added, new diagnostic concepts to be created, new prognostic variables to consider, new forms of treatment, new ways to evaluate responses, and new ways of storing patient instances so that they contribute to ease and versatility in diagnosing and treating. With a consistent structure built into one's storage system, the adding, deleting, and revisions become easier.

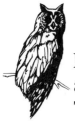

Exercises in Organization of Knowledge and Experience for Diagnostic and Treatment Decision Making

Set 1 □ Organize Diagnostic Concepts Presently Held in Long Term Memory

1. Select a diagnostic content area that interests you—one you encounter in your clinical practice and on which you feel you already have some information. If you wish, focus it by limiting it to a particular age group (e.g., neonates, adolescents, adults, people over 70) or a particular form of clinical specialty or pathology (e.g., perinatal, dementia, oncology, head and neck surgery, rheumatoid arthritis in children).

Without consulting any books, use the outline on pp. 176–177 to retrieve what you know about this diagnostic-treatment concept. Don't worry about using professionally "correct" words or full sentences—just capture your thoughts in words as they occur (try using a thesaurus to enable you to be as precise in your meaning as you can be). Do not try to do it in one sitting. Spend a block of time on it, sleep on it, think about it, and then come back and add to it. Use one page for each heading so that you can add or edit comfortably. Think about the patients you have encountered where this phenomenon was at risk or was occurring. What did you see? What did you hear? What did you notice? Use your knowledge from these encounters as well as that which you learned in lectures or reading.

2. Recall as many clinical and nonclinical instances as you can that contribute to any segment of your diagnostic concept. Some will illustrate risk factors, others manifestations, some a range of underlying dynamics, others prognostic variables, complications associated with the problem or treatment, treatment options that worked or did not work and responses to treatment. Write them down using first names or some identifying feature and the core situation. For example:

Underlying dynamics for nonparticipation in a treatment regimen:

John: Didn't believe that he was hypertensive (denial).

Mary: Too preoccupied with caring for young children to admit to her own need for care and to take time to do it.

Sarah: Hands too gnarled to self-administer insulin injections.

Juan: Believed currandero provides more effective health care than Western medicine.

Peter: Lived in a dirty room with a shared toilet and no laundry facilities—vulnerable to infections and had repeated ones. No money or desire to live elsewhere.

Tara: Drug use had priority over any health consideration.

Felice: Husband refused to give permission for self-breast examination, mammogram, or pap smears.

Carl: Lived 60 miles from clinic and had no transportation to come in for checkups.

Joan
& Sam: Believed that sufficient faith in God would heal their child's pneumonia and that calling in health care workers would show a lack of faith and cause the child to die.

Learning to gain access to the "video" part of your memory library and using it to support content in the "book" portion is important in breathing life into otherwise sterile theoretic concepts. Actual instances also tend to add to the variability that can be considered when one uses the concept.

3. **After** you feel that you have retrieved as much as you can recall, look at what you have written. Where is it rich, practical, scientifically supported? In what areas do you need to develop it further? Talk with or show it to your colleagues or ask for their ideas or experiences with any part of the diagnostic concept. Compare and edit.

4. Consult specialty texts and journals to see how others have conceptualized the subject. Review literature in fields other than the one you selected, e.g., the loneliness of psychotic individuals is described in psychiatric literature somewhat differently than it is in literature discussing it from a nonpsychiatric point of view. For examples consistently using the outline to describe a variety of phenomena (e.g., anorexia, asthenia, constipation, diarrhea, dying, dyspnea, eating difficulties, fatigue, hope, acute or chronic pain, role relationships, sexuality, social isolation), see *The Cancer Experience: Nursing Diagnosis and Management* (Carnevali and Reiner, 1990). *Nursing Diagnosis: Application to Clinical Practice,* 3rd ed. (Carpenito, 1989) offers diagnostic concepts using the NANDA categories and consistently gives: description of the phenomena, risk factors, major and minor characteristics (manifestations), outcome criteria (evaluation) and treatment guidelines for 110 different diagnostic concepts.

5. Refine your concept as needed. Then put your currently written concept in a labeled file folder, together with any copies you have made of supporting literature. Move on to another. You will find that the process is progressively easier as you develop patterns of thinking in terms of the parts of the diagnostic concepts.

If you find the structure offered in this chapter cumbersome or inefficient, modify it or develop your own.

Set 2 □ Building New Diagnostic Concepts

1. As new diagnostic concepts are introduced in classes, reading, and clinical experiences, restructure them so that they fit into the structure you have set up for your library and individual "books" and "videos." As you care for patients and use these concepts, purposefully store new material or modifications in the structure. As you encounter patient instances, think of the "title" you would use to retrieve them.

References

Bruerra E, MacDonald RN: Asthenia in patients with advanced cancer. *Journal of Pain and Symptom Management* 3:9, 1988.

Carnevali D, Reiner A: *The Cancer Experience: Nursing Diagnosis and Management.* Philadelphia: J.B. Lippincott, 1990.

CARPENITO L: *Nursing Diagnosis: Application to Clinical Practice*. 4th ed. Philadelphia: J.B. Lippincott, 1991.

GORDON M: *Nursing Diagnosis: Process and Application*. 2nd ed. New York: McGraw-Hill, 1987.

HAYLOCK P, HART L: Fatigue in patients receiving localized radiation. *Cancer Nursing* 2:461, 1979.

OREM D: A concept for self-care for the rehabilitation process. *Rehabilitation Nursing* 10(3):33–36, 1985.

PATRICK M, WOODS S, CRAVEN R, ROKOSKY J, BRUNO P: *Medical-Surgical Nursing: Pathophysiological Concepts*. 2nd ed. Philadelphia: J.B. Lippincott, 1991.

PIPER B, LINDSEY A, DODD J: Fatigue mechanisms in cancer patients: developing nursing theory. *Oncology Nursing Forum* 14:17, 1987.

RHOTEN D: Fatigue and the postsurgical patient. In Norris CM (ed): *Concept Clarification in Nursing*. Rockville, MD: Aspen Publishers, 1982.

ROY C, ROBERT S: *Theory Construction in Nursing: An Adaptation Model*. Englewood Cliffs, NJ: Prentice-Hall, 1981.

SCHMIDT H, NORMAN G, BOSHUIZEN H: A cognitive perspective on medical expertise: theory and implications. *Academic Medicine* 65:611–621, 1990.

THEOLOGIDES A: Anorexins, asthenins and cachectins in cancer. *American Journal of Medicine* 81:296, 1986.

THEOLOGIDES A: Asthenia in cancer. *American Journal of Medicine* 73:1, 1982.

8

Role Relationships Associated With Nursing Diagnosis and Treatment Planning

Diagnosis and treatment decisions obviously cannot occur without the individual nurse's mental activity, but neither can they become effective without interaction with others. Engaging in nursing diagnosis and treatment adds different requirements to nurses' interactions in almost all professional contacts. When nurses undertake delegated medical activities, they engage in one set of role relationships with patients, families, physicians, nursing colleagues, and others. When nurses assume primary responsibility and accountability for nursing diagnosis and treatment planning, a different set of role relationships comes into play.

Spheres of Accountability and Influence

Each health care professional, each patient and family member bring to health care diagnosis and treatment a particular perspective and expertise as illustrated in Figure 8-1. In addition to differences in perspective and expertise, each participant has an area of responsibility and accountability.[1] At basic levels of health care knowledge and skill, patients, families, and professionals are able to make judgments and decisions across disciplines without the services of professionals representing that field (this is illustrated in the diagram by the broken lines). For example,

> Individuals purchase over-the-counter medications in drug stores, supermarkets, or natural food stores without consulting either physician or pharmacist, and engage in both self-diagnosis and self-care decisions.

However, at higher levels of complexity, the perspective and expertise of a person trained and licensed to make discipline-specific judgments and provide treatment are usually needed. In areas of advanced knowledge and skills, it is much more difficult to move from one's own field of expertise to that of another (as indicated by the solid lines in Figure 8-1).

This diagram suggests that diagnoses and treatment decisions are identified by the health care domain within which the phenomena or situations fall, not the profession of the person making the judgment. Thus, when a nurse makes a diagnosis within the medical domain, it is a medical judgment because it concerns medical phenomena. It does not automatically become a nursing diagnosis merely because a nurse was the one to make it. For example:

> A nurse in a coronary care unit making a judgment that a patient is about to go into a cardiac arrest is making a medical judgment—just as if it were made by a physician.

---

[1]**Responsibility** addresses having an obligation to undertake an activity. **Accountability** addresses having to answer for one's decisions and actions.

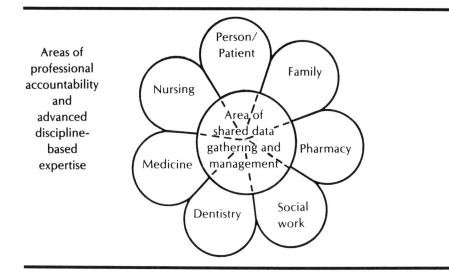

Areas of
professional
accountability
and
advanced
discipline-
based
expertise

FIGURE 8-1   Discipline-specific Perspectives and Spheres of Influence in Clinical Practice. From: Carnevali D, and Patrick M: *Nursing Management for the Elderly.* 3rd ed. Philadelphia: J.B. Lippincott, 1993. Used with permission

In the same way, persons in other health care fields make nursing diagnoses. For example:

A person who gathers data and makes a diagnosis involving a caregiver's difficulty in learning how to manage home care for a child on a respirator is making a nursing diagnosis—just as if it were made by a nurse.

It is the discipline-specific perspective and phenomena being diagnosed that determine the discipline label and ultimate accountability. Professionals in health care fields often cross discipline lines to make judgments and undertake actions. At the same time members of specific disciplines involved in a patient's care need to be certain that diagnoses and treatment plans in their own field have been appropriately and correctly made, whether done by a member of their own or another profession. For patients under their care, nurses are accountable for accurate, appropriate nursing diagnosis and treatment, regardless of which health care provider makes the decisions and offers the care.

If a patient or family place their health care into the hands of professionals in a particular discipline, ultimate accountability for the quality of the decisions and care rests with the professionals in that field. Thus, nurses may make judgments and decisions in the medical field and have accountability for reasonable standards of practice, but the patient's physician has ultimate medical accountability. When physicians or other health care workers make judgments and decisions in the nursing field and nurses are involved in the patient's care, then nurses have ultimate accountability for the quality of the nursing care the patient and family receive.

Each discipline's area of primary responsibility and accountability determines the role relationships members of that profession have with each other and with patients and their families.

Role Relationships when Nurses Make Judgments in the Medical Domain

When nurses cross discipline lines to make clinical judgments and take action, it is most frequently with medicine. There is no question that patient and family well-being requires nurses to make clinical judgments and decisions in the medical domain. Nurses are with patients in institutional, home, and community settings a great deal more of the time than physicians. There is also a long tradition and legal support for this part of nursing's role.

Role Relationships with Physicians

Nurses receive authority to make medical judgments and carry out treatments in several ways. It is a part of their role for which they receive extensive education. Institutional, agency, and clinical unit policies spell out the nature of nurses' responsibilities and accountability for functioning in the medical area with their clientele. Physicians' oral and written orders for individual patients or standard orders for groups of their patients determine nursing's responsibility to a physician for individual patients. In many settings physicians give wide latitude to nurses' judgments. They may order, for example:

Keep serum potassium between 3.5 and 5.

A variety of options for pain control, leaving it to nurse's judgment as to which will provide optimum analgesia given the ongoing nature of the patient's responses and requirements in daily living.

Nurses who are not licensed as nurse practitioners have specific role responsibilities in their relationships to physicians when they are functioning in the medical domain.[2] These are to:

■ Do case finding—that is, notice data on risks for pathophysiological or psychopathological problems or to observe signs and symptoms that such problems already exist and to **refer the patient to appropriate sources of medical help**

---

[2]In many states nurses certified/licensed as nurse practitioners are, by law, permitted to diagnose and prescribe treatment in the medical domain.

for further medical diagnosis and treatment (if the problem does not lend itself to self-management by the patient).

- Observe data about the patient's situation and responses as they are relevant to diagnosed medical problems and **report such data accurately and precisely, orally or in writing, in a timely manner to the physician who has current accountability for the patient's medical care.**
- **Carry out medical activities** that have been delegated to nursing personnel via institutional or agency policy, or by the physician's individual patient orders (incorporating the latitude of judgment that is accepted policy in the setting) **and to document and report** the activities that have been implemented.
- **Refuse to carry out medically prescribed actions** if, in the nurse's judgment, the prescribed activity is incorrect and question medical orders that are adjudged not to be in the patient's best interests or against the patient's legally specified directives.
- **Observe patient response to medical diagnostic or treatment activities and report such data accurately and precisely, orally and in writing, in a timely manner to the physician or take action without medical orders** if the patient's situation is of an emergency nature and report and document the action taken.
- **Make recommendations to the physician and negotiate about medical treatment** that would seem to be appropriate based on the nurse's clinical judgment about the patient's medical situation (often this involves symptom management or the patient's adjudged capacity to participate in particular medical activities at a given time).

In order to carry out these delegated medical functions as a part of their nursing role, nurses are required to have an adequate knowledge base and the expertise to make safe judgments and provide treatment correctly. And, because these are delegated medical functions, nurses have an obligation to provide the patient's physician with pertinent information about the patient and nursing actions taken in a timely manner. In many work settings, nurses are expected to take on increasingly complex medical judgments and complex treatments, requiring a high degree of knowledge and skills.

See *Exercise Set 1-1* for activities for self-analysis and contrast of role behaviors with physicians related to delegated medical tasks.

Role Relationships with Patients and Families

Functioning in the medical domain carries with it certain role relationships and responsibilities to patients and their families. In the area of medical practice the nurse has role obligations to patients and families to:

- Refer them to reputable sources of medical care thought to be compatible with patients' and families' health care needs (and values/beliefs when these are known).

- Teach them through words and actions what the nurse's role is in collecting medically oriented data and providing delegated medical care.
- Educate them, as appropriate, about their rights in relationship to medical care, e.g., the rights to a second opinion; to make known their wishes, values, and concerns; to negotiate about medical treatment; to seek medical care from a different source; to give informed consent; to refuse medical treatment that is recommended (Joint Commission on Accreditation of Hospitals, 1987).
- Support their belief and confidence in their physician and the medical care that is being prescribed where this is appropriate.
- Help them develop or use strategies to negotiate for medical care that fits with their values and situation.
- Provide them with information and support that enables them to use medical health care resources in a cost effective and satisfying manner.
- Provide them with information about appropriate, cost effective strategies for seeking other medical care options when this is their choice.

When nurses relate to patients and families within the portion of their role that involves responsibilities in the medical domain, they have obligations to the patient and family, and to the specific physicians who are involved in providing their medical care.

See *Exercise Set 2-1* for activities to explore role behaviors with patients and families associated with nursing responsibilities for delegated medical tasks.

Relationships with the Law and Third Party Payers

Nurses who are delivering delegated medical care have certain obligations and constraints associated with legal requirements and regulations of third party payers.

Legal Responsibilities

While state statutes may vary, nurses in general have legal responsibilities and obligations in two areas—to use their professional judgments in order to provide a reasonable standard of care and to keep physicians informed of their observations and actions orally and in writing.

Nurses are obliged to use currently available knowledge and a safe level of expertise in making judgments in the medical domain and in carrying out delegated medical activities. They are expected not to act blindly but to question and consider physicians' judgments, treatment decisions, and actions. If the patient situation dictates that nurses take immediate action without consulting a physician, they are expected to use sound clinical judgment and to promptly inform the physician of the action taken. When nurses make observations or carry out delegated medical activities, they are expected to document accurately and chronologically and to inform the physician in a timely manner (Cohn, 1991; Shanks, 1991).

Responsibilities to Third Party Payers

The major responsibility nurses have to third party payers in the delivery of medical care is to document the care given on the required forms. This is done for appropriate cost reimbursement and accounting purposes.

Role Relationships when Nurses Engage in Nursing Diagnosis and Treatment

When nurses engage in diagnosis and treatment planning within the nursing domain, they have full accountability for data collection, diagnosis, treatment decisions, and evaluation of patient/family response. This results in altered role relationships with patients and families, physicians, other nursing personnel, governmental agencies, and third party payers. The relationship with patients and families is not that of a physician surrogate but of a primary professional caregiver with full responsibility and accountability for judgments and care given within the nursing domain. Interactions with other nurses and nursing personnel are changed when a nurse assumes diagnostic and treatment responsibilities. Relationships with the law and with third party payers are not quite as clear as when nurses are delivering medical care, but there are some guidelines that apply.

Role Relationships with Patients and Families

When nurses function in the nursing domain they have role responsibilities to patients and families to:

- Teach by words and actions the specific perspective and expertise nurses will bring to both patient and family health care that is different from the medical care they receive.
- Help them differentiate between the kinds of problems and experiences they bring for nursing diagnosis and treatment and the kinds of problems and experiences physicians or other health care workers are prepared to address.
- Help them learn to provide data that will enable the nurse to make the most accurate, precise diagnoses and give the most therapeutic, cost effective, and satisfying nursing care possible.
- Teach by word and action that nurses have full professional accountability for the quality of their nursing diagnosis and treatment.
- Promote an appropriate level of confidence in their nurse's ability and willingness to address and manage phenomena and situations within the nursing domain.
- Support them in decisions to seek a different source of nursing diagnosis and treatment if the current relationship is not effective or satisfying. Help them make the transition in a cost effective and nontraumatizing way.

In an unspoken way, patients and families have always known that nurses provide health care different from that provided by physicians and other health care providers. With the advent of nursing diagnosis and treatment, these differences are being made explicit, and the changes in role relationships associated with nursing accountability are becoming clearer.

See *Exercise Set 1-2* for activities exploring role behaviors when the nurse is engaging in nursing diagnosis and treatment.

Role Relationships with Physicians

Neither nurses nor physicians have fully clarified and implemented the changes in nurse-physician role relationships when nurses assume full responsibility for nursing diagnosis and treatment planning (Stein, 1967; Stein, Watts, and Howell, 1990). In most situations, role relationships associated with nursing's independent functions are emerging. Some are based on individual negotiations or trust from long experience between selected physicians and nurses. Some are emerging as nursing unit or institutional policy.

In general, nurse-physician role relationships ideally become more *collaborative* when nurses assume diagnostic and treatment planning responsibilities. Thomas (1976) developed a two-axis model to describe interaction. One axis was designed **cooperation**—behavior designed to satisfy the concerns or needs of others, and the other axis was **assertiveness**—behavior undertaken to meet one's own needs or concerns (see Figure 8-2). In this schema:

Avoidance is	low assertiveness, low cooperativeness
Accommodation or appeasement is	low assertiveness, high cooperativeness
Competitiveness is	high assertiveness, low cooperativeness
Compromise is	moderate assertiveness and cooperativeness
COLLABORATION IS	HIGH ASSERTIVENESS AND COOPERATIVENESS

In other words, collaboration involves acting in ways to assure that nursing's professional needs are met but also having concern for the concerns of the other profession as well. In a study done in the early 1980s involving questionnaire data from 1,044 staff nurses and 536 physicians plus interviews with 264 nurses and 180 physicians, a *competitive* approach was found to be used by members of each group to resolve difficulties more than half the time. The primary area for disagreement was the patient's general plan of care. Joint problem solving (collaboration) was rarely seen (Prescott and Bowen, 1985). (Additional information about collaboration in nurse-physician relationships is described in an article by Baggs and Schmitt, 1988.)

Many physicians find it difficult to accept and accommodate to these shifts in role relationships (Styles, 1984; Stein, Watts and Howell, 1990). They have been taught

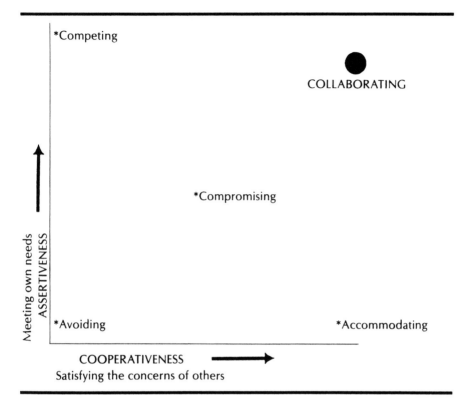

FIGURE 8-2   A Model of Collaborative Behavior. Adapted from Thomas K: Conflict and Conflict Management. In Dunnett M (ed): *Handbook of Organizational Psychology* Chicago: Rand McNally College Publishing, 1976, p. 900

by tradition, current education, and the threat of malpractice suits that they are fully accountable for everything that happens in the delivery of health care to their patients. Thus, they are reluctant to acknowledge an area of independent responsibility for nurses. Many physicians have no idea how the nursing perspective varies from their own in the delivery of health care. Often nurses themselves have created physician confusion by being unclear and variable in their descriptions and behavior. Additionally, physicians may have experienced inadequacies in some nurses' judgments and actions causing them to question the preparation and ability of all nurses to diagnose and to plan treatment in the nursing domain.

Regardless of the current state of affairs in nurse-physician relationships, there are some guidelines that apply when nurses engage in nursing diagnosis and treatment planning. Nurses in relating to physicians should be prepared to:

■ Assume full responsibility for the collecting of the nursing database; diagnosing, and prescribing treatment for phenomena and situations within the nursing domain; implementing that treatment and evaluating outcomes; and for document-ing these nursing activities in the patient's legal record.

■ Accept accountability for both successes and failures in nursing judgments and treatment.

■ Support judgments and decisions with a sound rationale, objectively and con-cisely presented, but to be open for new insights and changes.

■ Relate to physicians as professional colleagues, each with primary respon-sibilities for management of different areas of patient care.

■ Inform physicians about nursing data, judgments, and treatment, as needed, in order to achieve therapeutic, cost-effective integration of nursing and medical care that also satisfies the patient and family.

■ Present themselves and their information in such a way as to promote credibility and respect from physicians.

■ Assume personal responsibility in each physician encounter for enabling physi-cians to modify behaviors and attitudes that interfere with effective interdisciplin-ary delivery of nursing and medical care, e.g., use patient rounds or case con-ferences to consistently introduce and integrate the nursing perspective.

It can be seen from the above guidelines that interactions with physicians can be quite different when nurses are engaged in nursing diagnosis and treatment from behaviors associated with the delegated medical functions role.

See *Exercise Set 1-2* for self-analysis activities of behaviors with physicians associated with nursing diagnosis and treatment

As co-professionals assuming accountability for diagnosis and treatment in a separate domain, nurses are required to assume a more co-equal role. Not only must they be knowledgeable and expert in their own field, they must present themselves and their contribution in ways that create respect and acceptance. This involves one's appearance, body language, physical position in the group, pitch of voice, and language. Medical students are vigorously trained from the beginning to live with uncertainty and to support and defend their judgments and decisions when chal-lenged (Fox, 1957; 1980). Nurses with or without such basic training need to learn to support and defend their judgments in an equally competent, confident, and professional manner and to negotiate skillfully for patient's needs.

Not all nurses come into the nursing profession intending to undertake these professional relationships and their attendant stresses (Prescott, Dennis and Jacox, 1987). Not all nursing curricula provide the graduate with the prerequisite discipline-specific and interpersonal knowledge and skills to undertake the demands and challenges of interdisciplinary co-professionalism (Prescott and Bowen, 1985). Neither do all nursing service systems provide needed support for nurses to change traditional nurse-physician role relationships. Certainly, many individual physicians and medical groups within institutions and agencies have difficulty in understanding and supporting a complementary domain for nursing practice.

Nevertheless, patients and families need nursing care that is based on accurate nursing diagnosis and effective nursing treatment. Meeting patient-family needs depends upon nurses gaining command of power and resources to accomplish care-related activities. Nursing systems and individual nurses have obligations to modify physician-nurse reciprocal roles in such a way that both nursing and medical care can be appropriately provided.

Role Relationships with Other Nursing Personnel

Policies of facilities vary widely in the assignment of accountability for nursing diagnosis and treatment of individual patients.[3] In some settings a designated nurse has responsibility for planning patient care from admission to discharge or for a designated period of time. In other settings, diagnosis and treatment planning are integrated into unpredictably changing patient assignment, and these assignments can change in unpredictable patterns. Additionally, nursing diagnoses and treatment directives (sometimes called nursing orders) often do not carry the same weight as medical orders—nursing colleagues are free to follow them or not as they choose.

Nurses who are serious about planning individualized care for their case load of patients and families need to consider strategies for ensuring that the plans are implemented in a consistent and meaningful way. On an individual basis this may mean:

- Personally giving value to nursing diagnoses, treatment plans, and nursing directives.
- Behaving in ways that reflect value given, both in relationship to one's own plans and to implementing other nurses' plans.
- Creating diagnoses of sufficient accuracy and precision that others who read them gain insight into the phenomena or situations the patient is currently experiencing.
- Utilizing team or case conferences for shared formulation of nursing diagnoses and development of treatment plans.
- Writing treatment directives that are scientifically sound and so specifically written that they enable others, even those unfamiliar with the patient, to individualize care as the prescriber intended.
- Supporting written diagnoses and treatment directives verbally in assignment conferences or reports to other nurses.
- Seeking and using feedback about the effectiveness of one's diagnoses and treatment directives from those using them.

On a nursing unit or clinical service this may mean:

- Giving genuine value to nursing diagnosing and treatment planning, as contrasted to merely giving lip service to them.

---

[3]Assigned accountability for nursing diagnosis and treatment for a designated caseload of patients can be utilized with a variety of models of care delivery, such as primary nursing, team nursing, and case management. It is least effective when patient assignments are changed frequently and unpredictably or when tasks, rather than patients, are the focus for assignment.

- Negotiating for facility-wide/nursing unit norms and structure that make account-ability a feasible and consistent expectation.
- Negotiating for policies that provide for accountability of: 1) the individual nurse who diagnoses the patient and plans the care, and 2) those who implement the care as it has been planned.
- Seeking policies and norms that support rigor, precision, and accuracy in diag-noses and rational, specific treatment directives.

Nurses have been trained to accept a physician's authority to control their ac-tivities in delegated medical functions. It is not as comfortable to accept another nurse's control over one's perception of the patient's situation and one's nursing actions. At present, nurses who genuinely wish to have nursing diagnosis and treatment planning implemented may need to negotiate for acceptance of their plans with their nursing colleagues in addition to communicating the plans in writing.

See *Exercises Set 3* for activities related to communicating values.

Relationships with Accrediting Agencies, the Law, and Third Party Payers

Nursing leaders in governmental bodies, accrediting agencies, and professional organizations have played a major role in institutionalizing nurses' responsibility and accountability as diagnosticians and treatment planners in the nursing domain. Evidence of planned individualized nursing care is required by accreditors and inspectors of hospitals, long term care facilities, and home care. Failure to receive accreditation carries with it strong penalties, in finances and status. There is, there-fore, considerable pressure by administrators on nursing staff to present evidence that nurses are in fact engaging in diagnosis and treatment planning. Some state professional nursing licensure regulations now specify that patterns of failure to make appropriate and accurate nursing diagnoses and to give related nursing care can be reason for disciplinary action, even loss of licensure. The standards of the profession and health care accreditors as well as the statutes of state governing bodies, in turn, set the guidelines used by lawyers to determine reasonable prac-tices.

Concerns of institutions and agencies regarding lawsuits by patients have caused some to take defensive action by consulting with lawyers about language and practices in individualized nursing care planning. For example, in some institutions:

Using the words "risk for" may be seen as being less acceptable than "potential for." "Secondary to" may be seen as making a judgment as to direct causality and may not be as acceptable as the less strongly stated "related to."

There may be a policy that no spaces may be left blank on the nursing assessment form.

The same guidelines that pertain to documentation in the medical domain apply in the nursing domain. One should document accurately and in chronological order. Relevant strengths or normal responses as well as weaknesses and deficits should be noted. It may be wise to document each case as if it were going to be scrutinized in a court of law.

Sometimes these institutional mandates and guidelines create a perception among nursing staff that nursing care planning is done for administrators, accreditors, and lawyers rather than for the patient (much as students see care plans/case analyses as being done for the instructor, not a means of gaining skill for patient care). The "letter of the law" is met, care planning is documented as required, but the patient's need for individualized care becomes lost in the process. For example:

> A neonatal critical care unit has three predetermined nursing diagnoses for all preterm infants and their parents. The diagnosis for each infant is "impaired gaseous exchange R/T prematurity," and for each parent, "anxiety R/T baby's health status" and "knowledge deficit R/T inexperience with prematurity." There is a standard plan of nursing treatment for each diagnosis.

> In some settings general categories of diagnoses and standard plans of care are used in lieu of precise diagnoses and individualized treatment—or, only those diagnoses in a computer system and the associated nursing treatment may be used even though data may be present to permit more precise diagnosis and more specific nursing treatment.

In the current cost-cutting climate, it will be a challenge to achieve a relationship with the statutes, standards, and guidelines of government bodies, accrediting agencies, and legal professionals that still keeps the patient and family as the central focus for nursing diagnosis and treatment planning.

Relationships with Third Party Payers

When nurses engage in nursing diagnosis and associated treatment planning, their role relationships with third party payers are often characterized by frustration and struggle. Payment plans tend to be tied to medical diagnoses rather than the person's capability for managing self-care with the illness experience. Do nurses give emphasis to the delegated medical treatment that may be incidental in order to provide the crucial nursing services? Sometimes regulations as to who may receive financial support impedes patient well-being. For example:

> Some regulations of third party payers indicate that the persons receiving home care must be unable to drive their automobiles. Nurses see patients who realistically need home-based care but whose lives would be made easier by their ability to occasionally use their automobile. Do they turn a "blind eye" to infractions, seek to enforce the regulation, or report the infraction and thus terminate needed nursing services?

> Oxygen in the home is reimbursed on the basis of patient need demonstrated by designated blood gas levels, yet the experience of dyspnea that is relieved by oxygen is not always closely linked to arterial blood gas levels (Janson-Bjerklie, Carrieri and Hudes, 1986; Zerwekh, 1987; US Department of Health and Human Services, Health Care Financing Administration, Medicare Program, 1985).

With ongoing efforts to control health care costs, nurses may face increasing numbers of regulations that interfere with needed nursing services and patient's well-being.

Acute Care Settings.   Within institutional settings, nursing diagnoses and treatments often dictate that a patient remain in the hospital an additional day or two so that they can be prepared to take on the demands of self-care and the home environment. Diagnostic Related Groups (DRGs) and prospective payment make it difficult to find ways either to keep patients in long enough to insure capacity for self-care or to mobilize caregivers in the home setting to provide care until the patient becomes self-sufficient.

See *Exercise Set 4* for activities linking nursing diagnoses and treatment to discharge date and planning.

Long Term Care Settings.   In long term care a somewhat similar situation occurs related to keeping patients on units where there is sufficient staff to help chronically ill or older, fragile individuals maintain gains they have struggled hard to achieve. Usually, once these goals are achieved, patients are forced to return to units where staffing levels are lower and there is less time to provide the assistance needed for retention of higher levels of functioning.

Home Care Settings.   Third party payers support home care that requires medically-oriented therapy, even though the patient's and family's greatest need may be for nursing-oriented therapy. Nurses have become skilled in the use of language to document medical elements of the care required to maintain financial coverage so that desperately needed, but unsubsidized, nursing care can be "piggy-backed" on to it.

It may be that the merits of nursing diagnosis and treatment will become more fully recognized as research demonstrates cost effectiveness of nursing care based on an accurate diagnosis and rational treatment. It may be that funding will eventually be based on patient needs rather than a one-discipline perspective. If this is to occur, nurses will need to:

■ Demonstrate clearly, concretely, and in great numbers their nursing diagnostic and treatment expertise.
■ Relate to legislators and others who control funds in ways that show that this kind of care is cost effective.

Summary

It is not enough to think through and develop sharp, accurate diagnoses, appropriate prognoses, and therapeutic treatment, even though these are fundamental to effective nursing care. Beyond this is the requirement of interacting with others to implement and integrate nursing care into the patient's and family's health care gestalt. It is important to be able to interact with the system in such a way as to achieve credibility and recognition for the contribution nursing diagnosis and treatment make to patients' and their families' health and well-being. It is also necessary to persist in seeking ways to finance and obtain the resources that will permit effective nursing diagnosis and treatment.

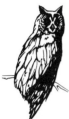

Exercises in Role Relationships Associated with Nursing Diagnosis and Treatment Planning

Set 1 ☐ Role Relationships with Physicians

1. Set your watchbird to notice your behavior, voice, and language as you interact with physicians while providing them with patient data or information about actions taken in the *medical domain*. Listen to yourself, note your body language, position, and voice pitch. Observe the physicians' responses.

2. Then set your watchbird to notice your behavior, voice, and language as you interact with physicians while presenting the *nursing perspective* on one of their patients (nursing diagnosis, prognosis, and treatment planning) as it integrates with medical planning. Listen to your tone of voice, your language; note your position, and your body language. Observe physician responses. Compare: 1) your behavior in the delegated medical component of your nursing role and in the primary nursing role, and 2) physician responses in each of the interactions. Were there any differences? Do your findings suggest any areas for change in either role? In any aspects of your own behavior (verbal, nonverbal)?

Set 2 ☐ Role Relationships with Patients

1. Set your watchbird to notice your behavior with patients and their families when you are functioning in a delegated medical role and as a nursing diagnostician and care planner. Specifically identify any differences you were able to discover (e.g., subject matter, language, tone of voice, expectations). Were there any differences? Do your findings suggest any areas for change?

Set 3 ☐ Behavior Communicating Values Held for Nursing Diagnosis and Treatment

1. Observe your behavior on the clinical unit as it reflects the value you assign to nursing diagnosis and treatment planning. Identify specific behaviors and the values that they could communicate to yourself and to others (e.g., how you talk

about them, priority and time you find to accomplish them, persons to whom you communicate them, degree of enthusiasm you exhibit).
2. Apply the same exercise to observing other nurses on the clinical unit. Identify specific behaviors and the values for nursing diagnosis and treatment planning they communicate to you. Do these behaviors have any impact on the quality of nursing diagnoses and treatment planning on the unit?

Set 4 □ Nursing Judgments
and Influencing of Discharge Planning

1. Select a patient on your unit who is on Medicare. Make nursing diagnoses and treatment plans associated with the individual's situation in assuming self-care responsibilities at the time of the designated discharge date. Gather data on the home environment (stairs, location of the bathroom and bedrooms, laundry facilities, telephone, heating, food-related facilities, transportation, as appropriate to the patients health status) and requirements in daily living (demands associated with self-care, medical treatments, and care of others). Gather data on the person's predicted functional capacities at time of discharge as they may affect self-care capacities within the home environment. Gather data on external resources to assist with managing the requirements of daily living.

Make a judgment as to whether the proposed DRG discharge date realistically permits this patient to manage daily living at home, given the environment, requirements, functional capacities, and external resources. If you have identified serious difficulties for the patient in managing at home, how would you present this to the physician or review committee in order to persuade them to give the patient another day or two of recovery? Role-play your presentation advocating a delay in discharge date. Record your presentation on audio- or videotape. Assume the role of the person who is charged with the responsibilities for approving the days of stay. Review the audio- or videotaped presentation. Critique the presentation in terms of its effect on you as administrator and on the decision you would make.

References

BAGGS J, SCHMITT M: Collaboration between nurses and physicians. *Image: Journal of Nursing Scholarship* 20(3):145–149, 1988.

CARNEVALI D, REINER A: *The Cancer Experience: Nursing Diagnosis and Management.* Philadelphia: J.B. Lippincott, 1990.

COHN S: Medical-surgical nursing legal principles. In Patrick M, Woods S, Craven R, Rokosky J, Bruno P (eds): *Medical-Surgical Nursing: Pathophysiological Concepts.* 2nd ed. Philadelphia: J.B. Lippincott, 1991, pp. 48–54.

FOX RC: The evolution of medical uncertainty. *Millbank Memorial Fund Quarterly/Health and Society* 58(1):1–49, 1980.

Fox RC: Training for uncertainty. In Merton RK, Reader G, Kendal PL (eds): *The Student Physician.* Cambridge, MA: Harvard University Press, 1957, pp. 207–241.

Janson-Bjerklie S, Carrieri V, Hudes M: The sensations of pulmonary dyspnea. *Nursing Research* 35:154, 1986.

Joint Commission on Accreditation of Hospitals. Bill of Rights Manual. Chicago, 1987.

Prescott P, Bowen S: Physician-nurse relationships. *Annals of Internal Medicine* 103:127–133, 1985.

Prescott P, Dennis K, Jacox A: Clinical decision making of staff nurses. *Image: Journal of Nursing Scholarship* 19:56–62, 1987.

Shanks SR: Legal issues in psychiatric mental health nursing. In McFarland G, Thomas M: *Psychiatric and Mental Health Nursing: Application of the Nursing Process.* Philadelphia: J.B. Lippincott, 1991, pp. 933–942.

Stein L, Watts D, Howell T: The doctor-nurse game revisited. *New England Journal of Medicine* 322(8):546–549, 1990.

Stein L: The doctor-nurse game. *Archives of General Psychiatry* 16:699–703, 1967.

Styles M: Reflections on collaboration and unification. *Image: Journal of Nursing Scholarship* 16:20–21, 1984.

Thomas K: Conflict and conflict management. In Dunnett M (ed): *Handbook of Organizational Psychology.* Chicago, IL: Rand McNally College Publishing, 1976.

US Department of Health and Human Services, Health Care Financing Administration, Medicare Program. Coverage of oxygen use in a patient's home. *Federal Register* 50:13742, 1985.

Zerwekh J: Comforting the dying dyspneic patient. *American Journal of Nursing* 87:66, 1987.

9

Professional Growth in Diagnostic Expertise and Decision Making for Nursing Treatment

It is not enough to gain basic initial competence in diagnosis and treatment planning. Maintaining and increasing these competencies is important to professional practice. It is a career-long necessity. The challenges and tasks needed to maintain clinical excellence in diagnosis and treatment planning vary at different stages of one's career. The areas for maintaining or increasing one's expertise tend to be the same, but the tasks involved can change over time as one spends more time in clinical practice.

Challenges at Different Career Stages

Variations in the tasks associated with attaining greater expertise in diagnosis and treatment decisions are shaped by a variety of factors occurring at different stages in a nursing career. Some of these include the status of:

- knowledge of the nursing perspective;
- knowledge and skills in diagnosing, making prognostic judgments and decisions regarding treatment in the nursing domain;
- knowledge of professional role and expertise in role requirements and role relationships;
- a rapidly changing theoretical and clinical knowledge base available for use in clinical practice;
- the command of language needed to describe data, diagnose, and prescribe treatment;
- clinical experience—amount, nature, clinical areas;
- psychomotor and interpersonal skills;
- values and accepted ethical guidelines associated with diagnosis and treatment planning;
- insight and personal criteria for self-evaluation of observation skills, critical thinking, decision making, and communication associated with nursing diagnosis and treatment planning;
- openness to change.

All of these determine the nature of personal work nurses need to engage in to maintain and upgrade diagnostic and treatment planning skills.

Challenges for the Nursing Student

The task of becoming initially competent in diagnosis and treatment planning looms large for the nursing student. There is so much to learn, and almost all of the elements in any nursing curriculum are essential to learning diagnosis and treatment planning. The list of basic requirements for initial competence in diagnostic and treatment planning include:

- A clear idea of the phenomena that are diagnosed and treatment modalities that are used in the nursing field.
- A structure or system for storing theoretical-clinical knowledge and patient instances to facilitate retrieval for nursing diagnosis and treatment planning.
- A command of discipline-specific language sufficient to influence clinical observation, thinking, and verbal and written communication. A valuing of words as nursing's "tools of the trade."
- Theoretical knowledge of normal human developmental tasks and age-related functioning as well as human pathology its prevention and treatment.
- An appreciation of the way in which knowledge from biological and social sciences and humanities are woven into the foundation for nursing diagnosis and treatment planning and how this knowledge is used in clinical practice.
- Ability to translate theoretical into clinical knowledge through repeated application in as wide a range of situations as is feasible.
- Psychomotor and interpersonal skills associated with nursing data collection and treatment implementation.
- Transformation of the problem solving process learned in earlier education and living into the diagnostic observation, thinking, and planning demanded by professional practice.
- Integration of the concept of prognosis with the concept of goals in order to produce realistic outcome expectations and treatment plans.
- Standards of excellence for diagnosis and treatment planning.
- Understanding and personal integration of the values and ethics associated with nursing diagnosis and treatment.
- Working knowledge of the professional role requirements and relationships associated with engaging in diagnostic and treatment planning behavior with patients, families, groups, and professional colleagues.
- Knowledge of body language, voice, and behavior needed to communicate confidence in one's judgments and decisions.
- Acceptance of responsibility and accountability for judgments and decisions made and strategies for managing the associated stresses.

These learning areas are usually incorporated into the basic curriculum that prepares nurses to assume the responsibilities of the beginning clinician. Varying lengths of programs, emphases, and differing approaches to clinical experience will determine how well these initial challenges are met and how prepared the graduate is to assume responsibility for nursing diagnosis and treatment planning in day-to-day practice.

Challenges for the Beginning Clinician

Even if all of the learning listed above is accomplished to some degree in the basic program, there are important challenges facing nurses as they engage in diagnosis and treatment planning in day-to-day practice. Carrying out these activities as an employee in the busy, distracting environment of the work setting with a larger case load creates different demands from those of a clinical course in a basic education program. Meeting the challenges of this transition from school to work environment effectively is important to continued effectiveness in nursing diagnosis and treatment planning. These challenges include:

- Acquisition of more theoretical knowledge, particularly that associated with nursing diagnosis and treatment of health problems of patients and families in the nurse's case load.
- Enriching of theoretical knowledge base with clinical knowledge and systematically storing patient-family instances for use in subsequent diagnosis and treatment planning.
- Storing knowledge and experiences in a system of diagnostic-treatment concepts, modifying and refining them as experience and knowledge grow.
- Increasing skill in observation as awareness grows of the complexity of the responses and situations to be diagnosed and the subtlety and variability of some manifestations of both potential and actual problems.
- Sharpening one's focus for nursing diagnosis and treatment in order to sustain a nursing perspective in the midst of the demands of delegated medical care for attention, time, and energy.
- Increasing the conciseness of one's thinking and communication.
- Learning to use words with the same sharpness and precision with which a skilled surgeon uses a scalpel.
- Learning to find the common denominator in a patient's multiple problems so as to make fewer and more integrated diagnoses and treatment plans.
- Increasing the speed and efficiency with which nursing data are collected, diagnoses and prognoses are determined, and treatment plans are made.
- Learning to time data collection, diagnosis, and treatment planning to when patient and family are available.
- Learning the working values and norms surrounding nursing diagnosis and treatment planning in the work setting. If there are differences between the system's values and personal values, finding a positive way to reconcile them.
- Increasing effectiveness and confidence in communicating nursing judgments, diagnoses, prognoses, and treatment plans to patients, families, community members, nursing colleagues, physicians, and other health care workers.
- Establishing a pattern for regular, purposeful, personal activities to promote ongoing development of diagnostic and treatment planning skills.

It can be seen that challenges in the early stages of one's nursing career are at least as demanding as those in the basic education program. There is still so much to be learned in both the theoretical and practical domains. Distractions of the busy work environment and multiple stressors and demands can make orderly development difficult.

Earlier, there were faculty members to offer some basic guidance to learning, and grades served as a prod. Now the responsibility for planned growth rests much more with the individual nurse. Patient and family encounters, contacts with other nurses (including nursing mentors if one is fortunate), and with physicians and other health care workers are one's learning opportunities. One can learn from them haphazardly and incidentally, or one can have a more orderly plan, so that one not only delivers the nursing care but grows in some self-directed ways as well.

Challenges for the Experienced Nurse

For experienced nurses the challenges are different. At present, the level of skill and comfort with nursing diagnostic, prognostic, and treatment planning activities can vary widely. Some nurses were not exposed to these skills in their earlier education and find it difficult to incorporate them in ongoing practice (Jakob, 1989).[1] Many are most comfortable working with clinical judgments and treatment within the medical domain. Others have learned particular approaches to diagnosis and treatment planning and feel most comfortable using only those. Still others are quite free-wheeling in their style of diagnosing and treating, venturing out in a variety of ways. In level of skill, comfort, and style, experienced nurses vary in their approach to nursing diagnosis and treatment decision making.

On the other hand, experienced nurses have much in common. A body of nursing knowledge has already been taken in and stored according to some pattern or system. That knowledge also has been used, modified, and refined in clinical situations. Patterns and skills of observation, data collection, and information processing have been established. Role expectations about patients' and family's participation in diagnosis and treatment planning are in place. Patterns of thinking and acting in the nursing role are usually well developed and comfortable.

Clinicians who are functioning in a familiar field and environment tend to use established scripts and task patterns as a way of carrying out everyday clinical encounters and tasks. These become the words and behaviors that are used almost automatically (Shank and Abelson, 1977; Gambrill, 1990).

Experienced nurses have essentially accomplished many of the tasks of the beginning nurse (with the possible exception of having learned the skills of diagnosis and treatment planning) and have developed patterns of thinking, working, and relating in ways that are generally compatible with the norms of the work setting. Both for those who understand the processes of diagnosis and treatment planning and those who do not, many of these activities are carried on with much less awareness than in earlier stages. These established patterns, which permit experienced nurses to function smoothly and effectively without having to be conscious of every thought or activity, may create difficulties in examining their diagnostic and treatment planning expertise. It is hard to gain insight into one's practices when they are carried on automatically.

---

[1]For nurses who have not had the opportunity to develop skill and comfort with the diagnostic process, the content in the earlier chapters of this book and the exercises should prove helpful.

Among experienced nurses, several general barriers exist for ongoing development in the areas of diagnostic thinking and treatment decision making. These may include inability to put "automatic" patterns of thinking into words; unrealistically high self-expectations even with a new task; fear of failure; lack of confidence; unwillingness to assign time for self-directed professional growth in the area of nursing diagnosis and treatment planning; unwillingness to disrupt comfort with present practice patterns; and satisfaction with present practice patterns.

The first challenge for experienced nurses is to become more aware of current patterns of practice. This probably cannot be done as a gestalt but needs to be approached one facet at a time. One approach is to set up a series of questions as a basis for gaining current self-knowledge. For example:

What do I think are my current working values associated with nursing diagnosis and treatment planning? Remember, these are working values, not necessarily ideal, e.g., one may have an ideal belief, but in practice have many, few, or no exceptions. "I believe the patient and family should be active participants in development of their nursing diagnoses and treatment plans except when. . . ." "I believe that nursing diagnoses have high priority when . . . and low priority when. . . ." "I believe that my treatment directives should carry equal weight with medical orders," or, "I believe that nursing treatment plans are written to satisfy quality assurance and accreditation criteria but not necessarily to affect patient care."

This list will be a personally held one, so it is both safe and essential to be honest even if the values are not the "politically correct" ones espoused by administration. These are data, *neutral* data, and therefore they should represent what is real and valid for you in your current practice.

Having completed this initial list of values and beliefs in as honest a way as possible, determine how to test whether your behavior/activities/attitudes honestly reflect these values and beliefs as stated. Tell your "watchbird" what to look for in your activities for this shift. For example:

How soon after contacting a patient or family member do I begin to focus on the nursing perspective for diagnosis and treatment?

In what proportion of my encounters with patients and families is the nursing perspective a focus?

Do I collect a nursing database because it is required by the institution or because I know the patient needs my nursing judgments to be based on these data?

Am I willing to deviate from the nursing history form if the patient's situation dictates a different focus?

Is the development of nursing diagnoses and treatment plans the "busy work"

I do when the "real work" is done or do I genuinely see them as essential to ongoing nursing care and to patient and family well-being?

Do I communicate my diagnoses and treatment plans to other nurses, to physicians, and to patients and families as if I value them? Specifically, how do my activities, words, and body language communicate these values?

What are my values associated with patient and family participation in the diagnostic and treatment planning process?

The use of a watchbird that is visualized externally to the nurse may assure collection of more objective data. It is important to focus the watchbird's data gathering on one question at a time and remain with that focus for a period of time long enough to get a fair sampling of behavior. If merely focusing on an area causes the behavior to change, consider the before and after. Once the watchbird has collected a usable sampling of activities, compare the data to the written list of values and beliefs, then edit it to make it fit with what the working value really is. If the revised working value is what the nurse wants, then nothing more need be done. If the final working value is unsatisfactory, then it can serve as a basis for reflection on what is desired and what changes in nursing behavior, attitudes, and activities are needed. Finally, experiment with the new behaviors.

An exercise in attaining greater self-knowledge and making changes when written out in this way seems like a laborious task. In actual time taken, it is not so overwhelming. Setting one's thoughts to focus on an area can be done while engaging in off-duty routine activities that don't require too much thinking. Once the process has been started, it tends to be maintained. Of course, extra time is needed to write the statements and to revise them.

Once one area of self-knowledge associated with diagnosis and treatment planning has been addressed and there is a sense of current completion, one can move on to another area. The earlier example dealt with values. For a change of pace one might then turn to a knowledge-oriented facet of practice. (Seek variety. It is important to keep these professional developmental tasks from becoming boring.) For example:

What are the nursing diagnostic-treatment concepts that I use most frequently? (identify specifically)

Is it possible that my range of available concepts for my case load is too narrow and that I am missing diagnoses because of this? For example, do I need diagnostic concepts related to cultural differences associated with my patients' health care practices? Are my patients and families experiencing losses in function, appearance, lifestyle—should I be using a concept of grief? Are usual roles and role relationships being disrupted in ways that make adjustments difficult for the patient, caregiver, or family—do I need to give more attention to the diagnostic concept of role? Does the disease or its treatment affect sexuality—do I have usable diagnostic and treatment concepts available for this?

Another approach would be to select one diagnostic concept that is either frequently used or changing and to refurbish it. For example:[2]

How long has it been since I reviewed the current literature on this concept?

How can I organize and sharpen this concept in terms of the recognition features, risk factors, and manifestations? Have I incorporated any new risk factors or manifestations from my clinical experience or discarded any that do not seem to apply? Moved any from the minor to major status based on frequency and importance? Determined particular manifestations that should not be found if selected diagnoses in this category are to apply? Discovered any muted, disguised manifestations?

Is there any new knowledge or research-associated findings on the underlying dynamics?

What are the diagnostic areas I currently associate with this diagnostic concept? Have any others occurred among patients that should be added?

What linkages have I made to other related concepts that tend to yield alternative diagnostic explanations or related diagnoses? Have they been useful? Have I looked to other diagnostic concepts with any patients who had problems within the original concept? Were they useful? Should stronger linkages be built between them in my memory?

Have I done any work on prognostic patterns, outcomes, or variables associated with this concept? What have I learned about each of these from my clinical experience with patients or families who have problems associated with this diagnostic concept? Do I need to add this section to my concept or modify the existing information by changing any of the patterns, outcomes, or variables?

What is the range of treatments for each of the diagnostic areas? How effective have they been? Is there any new knowledge concerning treatment for these diagnostic areas? How can I use my patient-family experiences to refine or expand my treatment options?

Have my criteria and strategies for collecting evaluation data on responses to treatment been on target and effective? Are there other sources of data on response that have arisen among my patients? Has the planned timing for collecting response data been appropriate? Is the language for describing response to treatment sufficiently precise qualitatively and quantitatively? How do I enable patients and families to provide data and make sound evaluative judgments?

Learning experiences described at the end of many of the chapters in this book also offer examples of other activities that may be undertaken to gain self-knowledge of

---

[2]For samples of a variety of diagnostic and treatment concepts, see Carnevali D, Reiner A: *The Cancer Experience: Nursing Diagnosis and Management.* Philadelphia, PA: J.B. Lippincott, 1990.

nursing practice and upgrade both knowledge and skills. For other ideas see "Additional Readings" at the end of this chapter.

Ongoing Tasks for Continuing Professional Development in Diagnosis and Treatment Planning

Nurses who wish to continue developing their diagnostic and treatment planning skills will address their ongoing efforts in several different areas. Generally, these fall into six interrelated areas:

- maintaining theoretical and clinical knowledge,
- tending one's long term memory filing system,
- noting one's current patterns of observation and information processing,
- increasing command of language,
- identifying working values,
- and developing role and role relationships.

Maintaining Theoretical and Clinical Knowledge

Obviously, knowledge in the health care fields, including nursing, is expanding daily—exploding might be a more precise description. Knowledge that nurses used in making nursing diagnoses and treatment planning at an earlier time often is replaced or modified. On the other hand, there is a need to judge the basis for new knowledge critically. Not every research project is a sound one and not everything that is published is worth accepting. Therefore, there are two dimensions to this task of staying abreast of the body of knowledge needed in order to diagnose and treat safely. Read and learn what is changing and what is not changing, then critically evaluate the basis or source for this new knowledge before accepting it completely. Certainly, testing in one's own practice the knowledge being offered (including this book), whenever this is possible, is a good idea. Engaging in vigorous discussion or deliberately debating both sides of the issue can improve both one's openness and evaluative skills.

Keeping up with the literature and the state of the art can be difficult in a busy nurse's life. Using colleagues who are recognized experts can be both interesting and efficient. Computer technology is improving access to literature in one's field. Conferences and continuing education classes also help.

Whatever the strategies used, nurses who engage in diagnosis and treatment planning have an obligation to remain abreast of the knowledge base and practices associated with areas they are diagnosing and treating. More general fields, such as ethical issues and cross-cultural content, are also important in diagnosis and treatment. Some systematic program and allocation of time is probably needed to maintain a current knowledge base from which to practice. Learning haphazardly only from whatever happens to come one's way is a weak substitute.

Tending One's Long Term Memory Filing System

As new theoretical and clinical knowledge and patient/family instances build up, there is some need to do updating and housekeeping in one's long term memory filing system. Diagnostic-treatment knowledge and clinical instances tend to be "filed" in terms of diagnostic concepts, phenomena, or situations, with linkages to other related material. As new knowledge is gained it needs to be stored in the "files" where it will be most useful. For example, new information about a particular cultural response to grieving might well be filed in the diagnostic-treatment concept of grieving but also with the particular culture represented. When patient or family experiences provide new etiology, risk factors, or manifestations for a particular diagnosis, prognostic variables, complications, or responses to treatment, the processing of this information and experience should lead to their being added to both the diagnostic-treatment concept in semantic memory and the patient and family instance file associated with that concept in episodic memory. When new research demonstrates that etiology/risk factors or manifestations are found to be incorrect and new ones are added, or when the possibility of describing them becomes more precise, the diagnostic-treatment concept needs to be modified accordingly. When new linkages or stronger linkages are found between diagnostic-treatment concepts, the processing should result in these linkages being strengthened. If it is found that previously accepted linkages do not exist, those linkages between diagnostic-treatment concepts should be removed.

As discussed in Chapter 2, very little information is believed to be lost from long term memory. The difficulty comes in gaining access to it, just as in any complex storage system. If the major high frequency or high priority diagnostic-treatment concepts used in a nurse's clinical practice are well organized and maintained, there may be better, quicker access to them when they are needed.

Noting One's Current Patterns of Observation and Information Processing

Self-knowledge is important in maintaining and increasing one's diagnostic and treatment planning expertise (Nickerson, 1986). Over time, changes can gradually take place. Some of these may reflect greater expertise; others may show a slipping of rigor and effectiveness or burnout. For example:

With pressures of increasing case loads or time constraints nurses may find themselves responding with:

- less tolerance for ambiguity;
- diagnoses that do not reflect uncertainty;
- diagnoses for which there isn't adequate supporting data;
- general diagnoses when there are data to support more specific ones;
- standard treatment plans increasingly used without planned individualization.

On the other hand, nurses may discover increasing skill and speed in identifying important data, in making clinical judgments, in making appropriately precise diagnoses, in making prognoses, in validating techniques, and in selecting therapeutic treatment options. There may be an awareness of gaining expertise in one area of specialization (e.g., neonatal care) while losing it in other areas where there is little opportunity for clinical practice (e.g., care of adults).

Increasing Command of Language for Precision in Diagnoses and Treatment Directives

Most nurses have not thought of words as crucial tools in the practice of nursing. Yet precise words are needed to adequately recognize and accurately describe data, to frame diagnoses, to differentially diagnose, to prescribe treatment, and to evaluate response to treatment. One needs words to communicate to oneself and certainly to others. With a rich vocabulary and the ability to use words as a reflection of the nursing knowledge base, a nurse is more likely to effectively describe, differentially diagnose, synthesize, and prescribe.

Constant alertness to the use of language is important in nursing. This can be done by listening to others describe patient data or situations and then seeking to find words that are more precise and accurate. It can be done by paying attention to one's own use of words and consistently seeking the best words until one becomes uncomfortable and dissatisfied with inexact language. An inexpensive, paperback thesaurus is invaluable in improving one's store of words.

Identifying Working Values Associated with Nursing Diagnosis and Treatment Planning

Working values are those that guide everyday choices, priorities, and actions. Sometimes they match ideals and sometimes they do not. For an individual nurse, it becomes important to be aware of the real, working values held concerning the activity of nursing diagnosis and treatment planning. Areas where values may be held and strategies for becoming aware of these values are discussed earlier in the chapter in the section on "Challenges for the Experienced Nurse."

Most nursing units also have informal, working values associated with the execution of nursing diagnoses and treatment planning. One can learn to recognize these in the same way that one studies personal values. For example:

What nursing diagnostic and treatment behavior is rewarded? What behavior is sanctioned?

What supports exist for diagnosis and treatment planning?

What focus for nursing diagnosis and treatment planning has the greatest acceptance?

How much conformity in format and structure is required? What is the response to departure from these formats and structures?

It is important to be able to identify areas where personal values and those of the work setting are congruent and where they are not as a basis for recognizing possible stress points and need for negotiation.

Developing Roles and Role Relationships Associated with Nursing Diagnosis and Treatment Planning

Nursing diagnoses and treatment plans are not developed and implemented in isolation. These activities involve the people being diagnosed and treated as well as those who will implement the care and those who will diagnose and treat health problems from another discipline's perspective (see Chapter 8).

A genuine awareness and pride in nursing's contribution to health care are essential to realistic implementation of nursing diagnosis and treatment plans. Confidence and assertiveness are also important. While there is no substitute for effective diagnosis and planning, diffidence and uncertainty, in presenting both oneself and one's diagnoses and treatment plans, can limit credibility that others place in them—even when the diagnosis and treatment plan are good.

There are opportunities to develop more effective professional skills in relating to patients, families, coworkers, physicians, and other professional colleagues around the activity of nursing diagnoses and treatment planning. There is also a need to negotiate for resources that make nurses' work in nursing diagnosis and treatment more feasible.

Summary

Reading a book such as this is one way to learn about the processes, constraints, and strategies involved in nursing diagnosis and treatment decision making as they are presently understood. Doing the exercises and adding personal clinical examples to those in the text offer even greater gains. Ongoing development requires maintaining some awareness of thinking and practice patterns, regular efforts to update one's knowledge base, attention to one's values and role relationships. It also requires self-confidence to engage in self-examination and an open attitude toward new ideas and personal change. While personal growth is sometimes described as painful, it also offers personal adventures and excitement as skills and expertise increase.

For patients, any increase in expertise in diagnostic skill and treatment decisions can have immediate and important benefits. Nursing diagnoses offer patients, families, and groups either opportunities or limitations, comfort or suffering, increased or decreased well-being. Given the benefits that accrue to both clientele and nurses, there are compelling reasons to seek to attain the highest level of expertise in diagnosis and treatment planning possible.

References

CARNEVALI D, REINER A: *The Cancer Experience: Nursing Diagnosis and Management.* Philadelphia: J.B. Lippincott, 1990.

GAMBRILL E: *Critical Thinking in Clinical Practice: Improving the Accuracy of Judgments and Decisions About Clients.* San Francisco: Jossey-Bass Publishers, 1990.

JAKOB D: Between a rock and a hard place: Slogging away while in transition. In Carroll-Johnson R (ed): *Classification of Nursing Diagnoses: Proceedings of the 8th Conference North American Nursing Diagnosis Association.* Philadelphia: J.B. Lippincott, 1989.

NICKERSON R: *Reflections of Reasoning.* Hillsdale, NJ: Erlbaum, 1986.

SHANK R, ABELSON R: *Scripts, Plans, Goals and Understanding: An Inquiry into Human Knowledge.* Hillsdale, NJ: Erlbaum, 1977.

Additional Readings

ASHTON P, WEBB R: *Making a Difference: Teachers' Sense of Efficacy and Student Achievement.* New York: Longman, 1986.

BARLOW D, HAYES S, NELSON R: *The Scientist Practitioner: Research and Accountability in Clinical and Educational Settings.* New York: Pergamon Press, 1984.

BRANDSFORD J, STEIN B: *The IDEAL Problem Solver: A Guide for Improving Thinking, Learning and Creativity.* New York: W.H. Freeman, 1984.

CHIRIBONGA D, JANKINS G, BAILEY J: Stress and coping among hospice nurses: Test of an analytic model. *Nursing Research* 32:294–299, 1983.

EDELMANN R: *The Psychology of Embarrassment.* New York: Wiley, 1987.

FLEMING D, FLEMING E, ROACH, K, OKSMAN, P: Conflict management. In Maher CA (ed): *Professional self-management: Techniques for Special Service Providers.* Baltimore, MD: Brooks, 1985.

GOETHALS G, RECKMAN R: The perception of consistency in attitudes. *Journal of Experimental Social Psychology* 9:491–501, 1973.

GREEN B, McCLOSKEY M, CARAMAZZA A: The relation of knowledge to problem solving with examples from kinematics. In Chipman S, Segal J, Glaser R (eds): *Thinking and Learning Skills,* Vol 2. *Research and Open Questions.* Hillsboro, NJ: Erlbaum, 1985.

HARMON G: *Change in View: Principles of Reasoning.* Cambridge, MA: MIT Press, 1986.

KOTTLER J, BLAU D: *The Imperfect Therapist: Learning from Failure in Therapeutic Practice.* San Francisco: Jossey-Bass, 1989.

NEURINGER A: Self-experimentation. *Behaviorism* 9:79–94, 1981.

ROKEACH M: *The Open and Closed Mind.* New York: Basic Books, 1960.

SCHLENKER B, LEARY M: Social anxiety and self-presentation: A conceptualization and model. *Psychological Bulletin* 92:641–669, 1982.

WATSON D, THARP, R: *Self-directed Behavior: Self-modification for Personal Adjustment.* 4th ed. Monterey, CA: Brooks/Cole, 1985.

WEISBERG R: *Creativity, Genius and Other Myths.* New York: W.H. Freeman, 1986.

A

NANDA Approved Nursing Diagnoses[1]

This list represents the NANDA approved nursing diagnoses for clinical use and testing (1990). Changes have been made in 15 labels for consistency.

Pattern 1: Exchanging

1.1.2.1.	Altered Nutrition: More than body requirements
1.1.2.2.	Altered Nutrition: Less than body requirements
1.1.2.3.	Altered Nutrition: Potential for more than body requirements
1.2.1.1.	Potential for Infection
1.2.2.1.	Potential Altered Body Temperature
1.2.2.2.	Hypothermia
1.2.2.3.	Hyperthermia
1.2.2.4.	Ineffective Thermoregulation
1.2.3.1.	Dysreflexia
*1.3.1.1.	Constipation
1.3.1.1.1.	Perceived Constipation
1.3.1.1.2.	Colonic Constipation
*1.3.1.2.	Diarrhea
*1.3.1.3.	Bowel Incontinence

[1]Reprinted with permission from the North American Nursing Diagnosis Association, St. Louis, MO, 1992
*Categories with modified label terminology

233

#New diagnostic categories approved 1990
**New diagnostic categories approved 1992

3.2.2.	Altered Family Processes
**3.2.2.1.	Caregiver Role Strain
**3.2.2.2.	High Risk for Caregiver Role Strain
3.2.3.1.	Parental Role Conflict
3.3.	Altered Sexuality Patterns

Pattern 4: Valuing

4.1.1.	Spiritual Distress (distress of the human spirit)

Pattern 5: Choosing

5.1.1.1.	Ineffective Individual Coping
5.1.1.1.1.	Impaired Adjustment
5.1.1.1.2.	Defensive Coping
5.1.1.1.3.	Ineffective Denial
5.1.2.1.1.	Ineffective Family Coping: Disabling
5.1.2.1.2.	Ineffective Family Coping: Compromised
5.1.2.2.	Family Coping: Potential for Growth
**5.2.1.	Ineffective Management of Therapeutic Regimen (Individuals)
5.2.1.1.	Noncompliance (Specify)
5.3.1.1.	Decisional Conflict (Specify)
5.4.	Health Seeking Behaviors (Specify)

Pattern 6: Moving

6.1.1.1.	Impaired Physical Mobility
**6.1.1.1.1.	High Risk for Peripheral Neurovascular Dysfunction
6.1.1.2.	Activity Intolerance
6.1.1.2.1.	Fatigue
6.1.1.3.	Potential Activity Intolerance
6.2.1.	Sleep Pattern Disturbance
6.3.1.1.	Diversional Activity Deficit
6.4.1.1.	Impaired Home Maintenance Management
6.4.2.	Altered Health Maintenance
*6.5.1.	Feeding Self Care Deficit
6.5.1.1.	Impaired Swallowing
6.5.1.2.	Ineffective Breastfeeding
**6.5.1.2.1.	Interrupted Breastfeeding
#6.5.1.3.	Effective Breastfeeding
**6.5.1.4.	Ineffective Infant Feeding Pattern
*6.5.2.	Bathing/Hygiene Self Care Deficit
*6.5.3.	Dressing/Grooming Self Care Deficit
*6.5.4.	Toileting Self Care Deficit
6.6.	Altered Growth and Development
**6.7.	Relocation Stress Syndrome

Pattern 7:   Perceiving

*7.1.1.	Body Image Disturbance
*7.1.2.	Self Esteem Disturbance
7.1.2.1.	Chronic Low Self Esteem
7.1.2.2.	Situational Low Self Esteem
*7.1.3.	Personal Identity Disturbance
7.2.	Sensory/Perceptual Alterations (Specify) (Visual, auditory, kinesthetic, gustatory, tactile, olfactory)
7.2.1.1.	Unilateral Neglect
7.3.1.	Hopelessness
7.3.2.	Powerlessness

Pattern 8:   Knowing

8.1.1.	Knowledge Deficit (Specify)
8.3.	Altered Thought Processes

Pattern 9:   Feeling

*9.1.1.	Pain
9.1.1.1.	Chronic Pain
9.2.1.1.	Dysfunctional Grieving
9.2.1.2.	Anticipatory Grieving
9.2.2.	Potential for Violence: Self-directed or directed at others
**9.2.2.1.	High Risk for Self-Mutilation
9.2.3.	Post-Trauma Response
9.2.3.1.	Rape-Trauma Syndrome
9.2.3.1.1.	Rape-Trauma Syndrome: Compound Reaction
9.2.3.1.2.	Rape-Trauma Syndrome: Silent Reaction
9.3.1.	Anxiety
9.3.2.	Fear

DEFINITIONS OF HUMAN RESPONSE PATTERNS,[1] OCTOBER 1989

Human Response Pattern	Definition	Human Response Pattern	Definition
Choosing	To select between alternatives: the action of selecting or exercising preference in regard to a matter in which one is a free agent; to determine in favor of a course to decide in accordance with inclinations	Exchanging	To give, relinquish or lose something while receiving something in return; the substitution of one element for another; the reciprocal act of giving and receiving
Communicating	To converse: to impart, confer or transmit thoughts, feelings or information, internally or externally, verbally or non-verbally	Feeling	In experience a consciousness, sensation, apprehension or sense: to be consciously or emotionally affected by a fact, event or state
		Knowing	To recognize or acknowledge a thing or a person,

[1] From Fitzpatrick JJ. Taxonomy II: Definitions and Development. In North American Nursing Diagnosis Association, Carroll-Johnson RM (ed). *Classification of Nursing Diagnoses: Proceedings of the Ninth Conference.* Philadelphia: J.B. Lippincott, 1991, p 25. With permission.

Human Response Pattern	Definition	Human Response Pattern	Definition
	to be familiar with by experience or through information or report; to be cognizant of something through observation, inquiry or information; to be conversant with a body of facts, principles, or methods of action, to understand	Relating	To connect, to establish a link between, to stand in some association to another thing, person or place, to be borne or thrust in between things
Moving	To change the place or position of a body or any member of the body; to put and/or keep in motion; to provoke an excretion or dischange, the urge to action or to do something, to take action	Valuing	To be concerned about, to care, the worth or worthiness; the relative status of a thing, or the estimate in which it is held, according to its real or supposed worth, usefulness, or importance; one's opinion of liking for person or thing; to equate in importance
Perceiving	To apprehend with the mind; to become aware of by the senses; to apprehend what is not open or present to observation; to take in fully or adequately		

Classification of Human Responses of Concern for Psychiatric Mental Health Nursing Practice[1]

1. HUMAN RESPONSE PATTERNS IN ACTIVITY PROCESSES
  1.1. Motor Behavior
      1.1.1.   Potential for Alteration
            *1.1.1.1. Activity Intolerance
            1.1.1.2.
      1.1.2.   Altered Motor Behavior
            1.1.2.1. Activity Intolerance
            1.1.2.2. Bizarre Motor Behavior
            1.1.2.3. Catatonia

[1]From O'Toole AW, Loomis ME: Revision of the phenomena of concern for psychiatric mental health nursing. *Archives of Psychiatric Nursing* 3(5):292–299. Appendix developed by M. Loomis, A. O'Toole, P. Pothier, P. West, and H. Wilson. With permission.
*Approved NANDA Diagnoses

<pre>
                  1.1.2.4.   Disorganized Motor Behavior
                 *1.1.2.5.   Fatigue
                  1.1.2.6.   Hyperactivity
                  1.1.2.7.   Hypoactivity
                  1.1.2.8.   Psychomotor Aggitation
                  1.1.2.9.   Psychomotor Retardation
                  1.1.2.10. Restlessness
          1.1.99. Motor Behavior Not Otherwise Specified (NOS)
   1.1. Recreation Patterns
          1.2.1.   Potential for Alteration
                  1.2.1.1.
                  1.2.1.2.
          1.2.2.   Altered Recreation Patterns
                  1.2.2.1.   Age Inappropriate Recreation
                  1.2.2.2.   Anti-Social Recreation
                  1.2.2.3.   Bizarre Recreation
                 *1.2.2.4.   Diversional Activity Deficit
          1.2.99. Recreation Patterns NOS
   1.3. Self Care
          1.3.1.   Potential for Alteration in Self Care
         *1.3.2.   Potential for Altered Health Maintenance
          1.3.3.   Altered Self Care
                 *1.3.3.1.   Altered Eating
                            1.3.3.1.1.   Binge-Purge Syndrome
                            1.3.3.1.2.   Non-nutritive Ingestion
                            1.3.3.1.3.   Pica
                            1.3.3.1.4.   Unusual Food Ingestion
                            1.3.3.1.5.   Refusal to Eat
                            1.3.3.1.6.   Rumination
                 *1.3.3.2.   Altered Feeding
                           *1.3.3.2.1.   Ineffective Breast Feeding
                 *1.3.3.3.   Altered Grooming
                 *1.3.3.4.   Altered Health Maintenance
                 *1.3.3.5.   Altered Health Seeking Behaviors
                           *1.3.3.5.1.   Knowledge Deficit
                           *1.3.3.5.2.   Noncompliance
                 *1.3.3.6.   Altered Hygiene
                  1.3.3.7.   Altered Participation in Health Care
                 *1.3.3.8.   Altered Toileting
         *1.3.4.   Impaired Adjustment
         *1.3.5.   Knowledge Deficit
         *1.3.6.   Noncompliance
          1.3.99. Self Care Patterns NOS
</pre>

2.6.2.2. Altered Concentration
2.6.2.3. Altered Problem Solving
2.6.2.4. Confusion/Disorientation
2.6.2.5. Delirium
2.6.2.6. Delusions
2.6.2.7. Ideas of Reference
2.6.2.8. Magical Thinking
2.6.2.9. Obsessions
2.6.2.10. Suspiciousness
2.6.2.11. Thought Insertion
2.6.99. Thought Processes NOS

3. HUMAN RESPONSE PATTERNS IN ECOLOGICAL PROCESSES
3.1. Community Maintenance
   3.1.1. Potential for Alteration
   3.1.2. Altered Community Maintenance
      3.1.2.1. Community Safety Hazards
      3.1.2.2. Community Sanitation Hazards
   3.1.99. Community Maintenance Patterns NOS
3.2. Environmental Integrity
   3.2.1. Potential for Alteration
   3.2.2. Altered Environmental Integrity
   3.2.99. Environmental Integrity Patterns NOS
3.3. Home Maintenance
   3.3.1. Potential for Alteration
  *3.3.2. Altered Home Maintenance
      3.3.2.1. Home Safety Hazards
      3.3.2.2. Home Sanitation Hazards
   3.3.99. Home Maintenance Patterns NOS

4. HUMAN RESPONSE PATTERNS IN EMOTIONAL PROCESSES
4.1. Feeling States
   4.1.1. Potential for Alteration
      4.1.1.1. Anticipatory Grieving
   4.1.2. Altered Feeling State
      4.1.2.1. Anger
     *4.1.2.2. Anxiety
      4.1.2.3. Elation
      4.1.2.4. Envy
     *4.1.2.5. Fear
     *4.1.2.6. Grief
      4.1.2.7. Guilt
      4.1.2.8. Sadness
      4.1.2.9. Shame
   4.1.3. Affect Incongruous in Situation

4.1.4.   Flat Affect
4.1.99.   Feeling States NOS
4.2.   Feeling Processes
    4.2.1.   Potential for Alteration
    4.2.2.   Altered Feeling Processes
        4.2.2.1.   Lability
        4.2.2.2.   Mood Swings
    4.2.99.   Feeling Processes NOS

5. HUMAN RESPONSE PATTERNS IN INTERPERSONAL PROCESSES

5.1.   Abuse Response Patterns
    5.1.1.   Potential for Alteration
    5.1.2.   Altered Abuse Response
        *5.1.2.1.   Post-trauma Response
        *5.1.2.2.   Rape Trauma Syndrome
        *5.1.2.3.   Compound Reaction
        *5.1.2.4.   Silent Reaction
    5.1.99.   Abuse Response Patterns NOS
5.2.   Communication Processes
    5.2.1.   Potential for Alteration
    *5.2.2.   Altered Communication Processes
        5.2.2.1.   Altered Nonverbal Communication
        *5.2.2.2.   Altered Verbal Communication
            5.2.2.2.1.   Aphasia
            5.2.2.2.2.   Bizarre Content
            5.2.2.2.3.   Confabulation
            5.2.2.2.4.   Ecolalia
            5.2.2.2.5.   Incoherent
            5.2.2.2.6.   Mute
            5.2.2.2.7.   Neologisms
            5.2.2.2.8.   Nonsense/Word Salad
            5.2.2.2.9.   Stuttering
    5.2.99.   Communication Processes NOS
5.3.   Conduct/Impulse Processes
    5.3.1.   Potential for Alteration
        *5.3.1.1.   Potential for Violence
        5.3.1.2.   Suicidal Ideation
    5.3.2.   Altered Conduct/Impulse Processes
        5.3.2.1.   Accident Prone
        5.3.2.2.   Aggressive/Violent Behavior Toward Environment
        5.3.2.3.   Delinquency
        5.3.2.4.   Lying
        5.3.2.5.   Physical Aggression Toward Others

5.3.2.6.   Physical Aggression Toward Self
      5.3.2.6.1.   Suicide Attempt(s)
5.3.2.7.   Promiscuity
5.3.2.8.   Running Away
5.3.2.9.   Substance Abuse
5.3.2.10.   Truancy
5.3.2.11.   Vandalism
5.3.2.12.   Verbal Aggression Toward Others
5.3.99.   Conduct/Impulse Processes NOS
5.4.   Family Processes
    5.4.1.   Potential for Alteration
      *5.4.1.1.   Potential for Altered Parenting
      *5.4.1.2.   Potential for Family Growth
    *5.4.2.   Altered Family Processes
      5.4.2.1.   Ineffective Family Coping
        *5.4.2.1.1.   Compromised
        *5.4.2.1.2.   Disabled
    5.4.99.   Family Processes NOS
5.5.   Role Performance
    5.5.1.   Potential for Alteration
    *5.5.2.   Altered Role Performance
      5.5.2.1.   Altered Family Role
        5.5.2.1.1.   Parental Role Conflict
        5.5.2.1.2.   Parental Role Deficit
      5.5.2.2.   Altered Play Role
      5.5.2.3.   Altered Student Role
      5.3.2.4.   Altered Work Role
    *5.5.3.   Ineffective Individual Coping
      *5.5.3.1.   Defensive Coping
      *5.5.3.2.   Ineffective Denial
    5.5.99.   Role Performance Patterns NOS
5.6.   Sexuality
    5.6.1.   Potential for Alteration
    5.6.2.   Altered Sexual Behavior Leading to Intercourse
    5.6.3.   Altered Sexual Conception Actions
    5.6.4.   Altered Sexual Development
    5.6.5.   Altered Sexual Intercourse
    5.6.6.   Altered Sexual Relationships
    *5.6.7.   Altered Sexuality Patterns
    5.6.8.   Altered Variation of Sexual Expression
    *5.6.9.   Sexual Dysfunction
    5.6.99.   Sexuality Processes NOS
5.7.   Social Interaction
    5.7.1.   Potential for Alteration

      *5.7.2.   Altered Social Interaction
            5.7.2.1.   Bizarre Behaviors
            5.7.2.2.   Compulsive Behaviors
            5.7.2.3.   Disorganized Social Behaviors
            5.7.2.4.   Social Intrusiveness
           *5.7.2.5.   Social Isolation/Withdrawal
            5.7.2.8.   Unpredictable Behaviors
      5.7.99.   Social Interaction Patterns NOS

6. HUMAN RESPONSE PATTERNS IN PERCEPTION PROCESSES
  6.1.   Attention
      6.1.1.   Potential for Alteration
      6.1.2.   Altered Attention
            6.1.2.1.   Hyperalertness
            6.1.2.2.   Inattention
            6.1.2.3.   Selective Attention
      6.1.99.   Attention Patterns NOS
  6.2.   Comfort
      6.2.1.   Potential for Alteration
      *6.2.2.   Altered Comfort Patterns
            6.2.2.1.   Discomfort
            6.2.2.2.   Distress
          *6.2.2.3.   Pain
                 6.2.2.3.1.   Acute Pain
               *6.2.2.3.2.   Chronic Pain
      6.2.99.   Comfort Patterns NOS
  6.3.   Self Concept
      6.3.1.   Potential for Alteration
      6.3.2.   Altered Self Concept
         *6.3.2.1.   Altered Body Image
         *6.3.2.2.   Altered Personal Identity
         *6.3.2.3.   Altered Self Esteem
             *6.3.2.3.1.   Chronic Low Self Esteem
             *6.3.2.3.2.   Situational Low Self Esteem
            6.3.2.4.   Altered Sexual Identity
                 6.3.2.4.1.   Altered Gender Identity
      6.3.3.   Undeveloped Self Concept
      6.3.99.   Self Concept Patterns NOS
  6.4.   Sensory Perception
      6.4.1.   Potential for Alteration
      *6.4.2.   Altered Sensory Perception
            6.4.2.1.   Hallucinations
                *6.4.2.1.1.   Auditory
                *6.4.2.1.2.   Gustatory
                *6.4.2.1.3.   Kinesthetic

                  7.6.2.4.5.   Visual
             *7.6.2.5.   Cerebral Tissue Perfusion
             *7.6.2.5.   Unilateral Neglect
             7.6.2.7.   Seizures
        7.6.99.   Neuro Sensory Processes NOS
7.7.   Nutrition
        7.7.1.   Potential for Alteration
             *7.7.1.1.   Potential for More Than Body Requirements
             *7.7.1.2.   Potential for Poisoning
        7.7.2.   Altered Nutrition Processes
             7.7.2.1.   Altered Cellular Processes
             7.4.2.2.   Altered Eating Processes
                  7.7.2.2.1.   Anorexia
                *7.7.2.2.2.   Altered Oral Mucous Membrane
             7.7.2.3.   Altered Systemic Processes
                *7.7.2.3.1.   Less Than Body Requirements
                *7.7.2.3.2.   More Than Body Requirements
             7.7.2.4.   Impaired Swallowing
        7.7.99.   Nutrition Processes NOS
7.8.   Oxygenation
        7.8.1.   Potential of Alteration
             *7.8.1.1.   Potential for Aspiration
             *7.8.1.2.   Potential for Suffocating
        7.8.2.   Altered Oxygenation Processes
             7.8.2.1.   Altered Respiration
                *7.8.2.1.1.   Altered Gas Exchange
                *7.8.2.1.2.   Ineffective Airway Clearance
                *7.8.2.1.3.   Ineffective Breathing Pattern
             *7.8.2.2.   Tissue Perfusion
        7.8.99.   Oxygenation Processes NOS
7.9.   Physical Integrity
        7.9.1.   Potential for Alteration
             *7.9.1.1.   Potential for Altered Skin Integrity
             *7.9.1.2.   Potential for Trauma
        7.9.2.   Altered Oral Mucous Membrane
             *7.9.2.2.   Altered Skin Integrity
             *7.9.2.3.   Altered Tissue Integrity
        7.9.99.   Physical Integrity Processes NOS
7.10.   Physical Regulation Processes
        7.10.1.   Potential for Alteration
             *7.10.1.1.   Potential for Altered Body Temperature
             *7.10.1.2.   Potential for Infection
        7.10.2.   Altered Physical Regulation Processes
             7.10.2.1.   Altered Immune Response

7.10.2.1.1. Infection
7.10.2.2. Altered Body Temperature
*7.10.2.2.1. Hyperthermia
*7.10.2.2.2. Hypothermia
*7.10.2.2.3. Ineffective Thermoregulation
7.10.99. Physical Regulation Processes NOS
8. HUMAN RESPONSE PATTERNS IN VALUATION PROCESSES
8.1. Meaningfulness
8.1.1.   Potential for Alteration
*8.1.2.   Altered Meaningfulness
8.1.2.1.   Helplessness
*8.1.2.2.   Hopelessness
8.1.2.3.   Loneliness
*8.1.2.4.   Powerlessness
8.1.99.   Meaningfulness Patterns NOS
8.2. Spirituality
8.2.1.   Potential for Alteration
8.2.2.   Altered Spirituality
8.2.2.1.   Spiritual Despair
*8.2.2.2.   Spiritual Distress
8.2.99.   Spirituality Patterns NOS
8.3. Values
8.3.1.   Potential for Alteration
8.3.2.   Altered Values
8.3.2.1.   Conflict With Social Order
8.3.2.2.   Inability to Internalize Values
8.3.2.3.   Unclear Values
8.3.99.   Value Patterns NOS

Eleven Functional Health Patterns[1]

Health-perception–health-management pattern Describes client's perceived pattern of health and well-being and how health is managed.

Nutritional-metabolic pattern Describes pattern of food and fluid consumption relative to metabolic need and pattern indicators of local nutrient supply.

Elimination pattern Describes patterns of excretory function (bowel, bladder, and skin).

Activity-exercise pattern Describes pattern of exercise, activity, leisure, and recreation.

Cognitive-perceptual pattern Describes sensory perceptual and cognitive pattern.

Sleep-rest pattern Describes patterns of sleep, rest, and relaxation.

Self-perception–self-concept pattern Describes self-concept pattern and perceptions of self (e.g., body comfort, body image, feeling state).

Role-relationship pattern Describes pattern of role-engagements and relationships.

---

[1]Gordon M. *Nursing Diagnosis: Process and Application. 2nd ed. New York: McGraw-Hill, 1987, p. 93. With permission.*

Sexuality-reproductive pattern Describes client's patterns of satisfaction and dissatisfaction with sexuality pattern; describes reproductive patterns.

Coping–stress tolerance pattern Describes general coping pattern and effectiveness of the pattern in terms of stress tolerance.

Value-belief pattern Describes patterns of values, beliefs (including spiritual), or goals that guide choices or decisions.

The Carnevali Daily Living ↔ Functional Health Status Model

While human responses or functional capacities can be viewed as separate entities, for nursing it seems reasonable to integrate them with requirements and supports of the situation within which the health experience occurs. This is the perspective of the Daily Living ↔ Functional Health Status Model. As shown in the arrow diagram in Figure E-1, daily living is seen to affect functional health status, and functional health status is seen to affect daily living. Each one is always viewed in relationship to the other, not in isolation.

For purposes of diagnostic and treatment thinking, it is useful to view the patient situation as an attempt to balance the requirements of daily living with the functional capacities and external resources for meeting those requirements as shown in Figure E-2. Note that balance may occur at very high levels, when functioning is excellent in most areas, adequate resources are available, and there is a supportive daily living environment. But balance may also occur at very low levels, when functioning is widely or seriously impaired, resources are not entirely adequate, and daily living is less than helpful. In most situations, patients and families will be seeking to maintain an acceptable, satisfying balance somewhere between these extremes.

Appendix E Figure 1

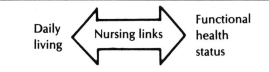

Domain for nursing diagnosis and treatment. (After Carnevali D, Patrick M. *Nursing Management for the Elderly*, 3rd ed. Philadelphia: J.B. Lippincott, 1993.

Appendix E Figure 2

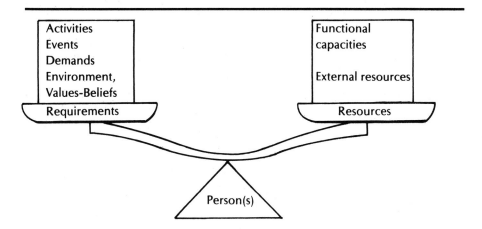

A model for nursing's data base, diagnosis, prognosis and treatment. Adapted from Carnevali D. Daily living and functional health status: a perspective for nursing diagnosis and treatment. *Archives of Psychiatric Nursing* 2(6): 330, 1988

Daily Living

In this model the **Daily Living** category is seen to be composed of five elements:

■ *Activities in Daily Living* consist of any activities of the diagnosed person that are relevant to the presenting health situation. This also can involve activities of others when these affect the patient. The activities may be *usual or unusual* for the person. Activities also have a time dimension. Relevant *past* activities are examined in terms of their effect on the person's emotional and physical response to present activities. *Present and future activities* are considered in terms of the functional capacities and external resources to carry them out. The *significance and meaning* of activities are also of concern when alterations may occur because of patient status or as a result of treatment.

■ *Events in Daily Living* are personal or health-related occurrences that affect or are affected by the presenting health situation, e.g., holidays, trips, anniversaries; or diagnostic test results, medical treatments, new diagnoses. Again, *past* events are examined for their effect on current responses (e.g., earlier chemotherapy, previous childbirth, etc.), and *present and future* events are contemplated in terms of functional capacities to undertake them. *Significance and meaning* of events to the patient and family also are important.

■ *Demands in Daily Living* arise from three sources–self, others, and one's possessions. They are expectations regarding activities, behaviors, choices, attitudes, values, priorities in daily living that affect emotional responses, choices, and behaviors. Self-expectations can incorporate body image, self-concept, obligations and role responsibilities, degree of independence. The source of others' expectations can be family, friends, and social or religious groups, health care professionals, employers, governmental bureaucracies. Possessions, such as living quarters, cars, animals, create demands. Demands can be in excess of, or less than, functional capacities. They also have real potential to conflict with each other. Times of transition in expectations and demands can create stress.

■ *Environment for Daily Living* is the specific context or milieu within which the daily living is taking place (institutional, home, work, school, the streets, etc.). Physical, microbial, sensory and interpersonal aspects of the environment are of concern. The priorities and specifics of concern depend upon the nature of the individual's or group's functional capacities, e.g., vision impairment creates one set of concerns about the environment, impaired immune systems another, restricted mobility still others.

■ *Values and beliefs:* Values are made up of the principles, priorities and relative worth of aspects of one's life and lifestyle. Beliefs are the mental acceptance of something as being "true." Nursing is concerned with those values and beliefs that play a part in the choices, feelings, actions, and interactions associated with the presenting health experience. Of concern are the values and beliefs of the patient or family but also of health care providers, personal caregivers, close friends, employers, etc. Examples of values and beliefs include beliefs about contagion, the right to choose health care freely, the right to die, the concept of illness as the result of wrong thinking or behavior, valuing of privacy, independence, one's roles and goals in life.

Functional Capacities

Functional Capacities are those internal resources available to the individual, family, or group to manage specific requirements in their daily living. They can include such internal resources as physical, mental, and emotional strength and endurance; cognitive capacities; sensory capacities; sexuality; mobility/flexibility; motivation; mood; capacities to take risks; capacities to make oneself understood; psychomotor and interpersonal skills.

External Resources

Managing the requirements of daily living effectively and with satisfaction often depends on more than one's internal resources. One's *external resources* or support systems can either enhance or diminish functional effectiveness. Resources external to the individual or family can include the architecture and amenities in one's housing, communication facilities, financial resources, housing, neighborhood, people, pets, services, supplies and equipment, technology, and transportation.

Nursing concerns itself with the resources that are needed, available, usable, and desired in the presenting situation.

Definition of Health Using the Carnevali DL↔FHS Model

Health, from the perspective of this model, could be defined as the achievement of balance between a person's daily living requirements and her/his functional capacities, plus external resources for sustaining the highest possible level of physical, psychosocial and spiritual well-being as well as a satisfying quality of life. Health, using this definition, could occur or be diminished at any level of wellness or illness, in any setting.

Nursing Diagnosis Using
the Carnevali DL↔FHS Model

Using the DL↔FHS model, nurses would diagnose and treat health-related problems associated with:

- The impact of functional health status on the individual's or family's capacities to maintain health and to manage the requirements of daily living and normal developmental tasks in an effective and satisfying way in the face of altered functional capacities.
- Any aspects of daily living that fail to promote health or produce added strains or demands on currently available or projected functional capacities or external resources.
- Difficulties in incorporating health behaviors or treatment regimens into daily living.
- Inadequate or inappropriate external resources that create barriers to effective and satisfying management of daily living associated with the presenting health situation.

Index